Mastering Keto Diet For Women Over 50

A Practical Guide To The Ketogenic Diet For Women Over 50 With Easy And Tasty Recipes And A Meal Program To Lose Weight, Boost Energy, Prevent Diseases And Stay Healthy

Josephine Berg

© Copyright 2021 - All rights reserved.

The content contained within this book may not be reproduced, duplicated or transmitted without direct written permission from the author or the publisher.

Under no circumstances will any blame or legal responsibility be held against the publisher, or author, for any damages, reparation, or monetary loss due to the information contained within this book. Either directly or indirectly.

Legal Notice:

This book is copyright protected. This book is only for personal use. You cannot amend, distribute, sell, use, quote or paraphrase any part, or the content within this book, without the consent of the author or publisher.

Disclaimer Notice:

Please note the information contained within this document is for educational and entertainment purposes only. All effort has been executed to present accurate, up to date, and reliable, complete information. No warranties of any kind are declared or implied. Readers acknowledge that the author is not engaging in the rendering of legal, financial, medical or professional advice. The content within this book has been derived from various sources. Please consult a licensed professional before attempting any techniques outlined in this book.

By reading this document, the reader agrees that under no circumstances is the author responsible for any losses, direct or indirect, which are incurred as a result of the use of information contained within this document, including, but not limited to, errors, omissions, or inaccuracies.

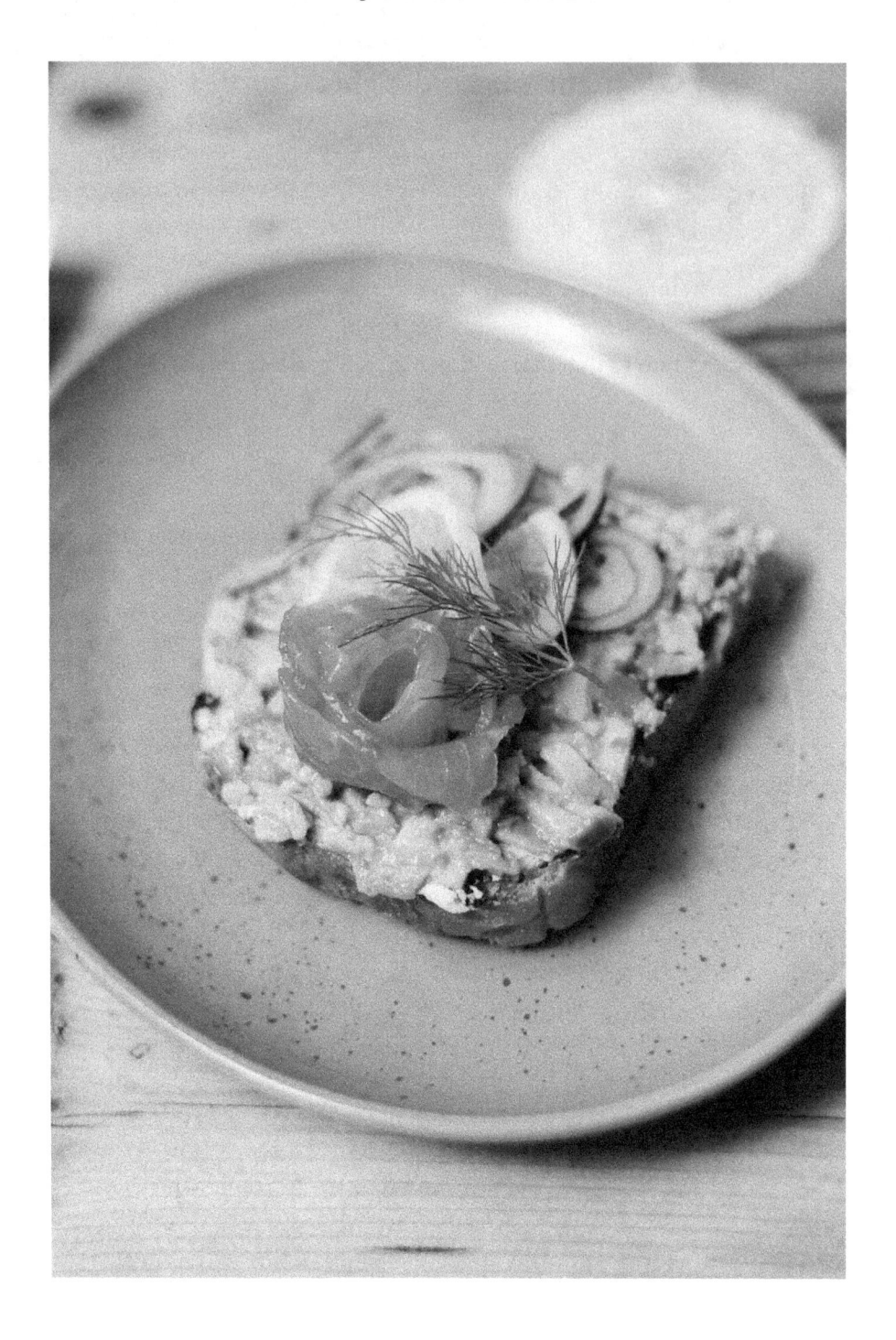

TABLE OF CONTENTS

INTRODUCTION 8

CHAPTER-1 10

    Is the Ketogenic Diet a Good Choice for Women Over 50? 10
    keto-fying your favorite foods 13
    A low-carb for women over 5 14
    Ketogenic food to consume 15
    foods you should stay away from 16

CHAPTER-2 OVER 50 OF OUR BEST KETO RECIPES 20

    Micronutrients are depleted by physical activity 21
    Non-nutritive, micronutrients, macronutrients, and macronutrients 22
    The best relaxation therapy 24

BREAKFAST RECIPES 26

    1. Everything Bagel Seasoned Eggs 26
    2. Beef & Veggie Hash 28
    3. Eggs & Spinach Florentine 30
    4. Walnut Granola 32
    5. Creamy Bacon Omelet 35

APPETIZERS AND SNACKS 38

    6. Tomatoes and Jalapeño Salsa 38
    7. Buttered Lobster and Cream Cheese Dip 40
    8. Prosciutto and Asparagus Wraps 42
    9. Low-Carb Cheesy Almond Biscuits 44

DINNER RECIPES 46

    10. Jamon & Queso Balls 46
    11. Bake for 13 minutes or until they turn golden brown and become crispy. 48
    12. Cajun Crabmeat Frittata 49
    13. Crabmeat & Cheese Stuffed Avocado 51

EASY PEASY RECIPES ... 54

14. Cheesy Brussels Sprouts Salad ... 54
15. Tomato Bites with Vegan Cheese Topping ... 56
16. Salami Cauliflower Pizza ... 57
17. Baked Cheese & Cauliflower ... 58
18. Spanish Paella "Keto-Style" ... 59

SALADS & SOUPS RECIPES ... 62

19. Modern Greek Salad with Avocado ... 62
20. Seared Rump Steak Salad ... 64
21. Cheesy Beef Salad ... 66
22. Pickled Pepper Salad with Grilled Steak ... 68
23. Parma Ham & Egg Salad ... 70
24. Chicken Salad with Gorgonzola Cheese ... 72

POULTRY RECIPES ... 74

25. Spicy Garlic Chicken Kebabs ... 74
26. Cheesy Chicken Dish With Spinach ... 77
27. Delicious Parmesan Chicken ... 79
28. Michigander-Style Turkey ... 82
29. Keto Chicken Casserole ... 84
30. Almond Chicken Cordon Bleu ... 87

PORK RECIPES ... 90

31. Chorizo in Cabbage Sauce with Pine Nuts ... 90
32. Hawaiian Pork Loco Moco ... 92
33. Pork Sausage Omelet with Mushrooms ... 94
34. British Pork Pie with Broccoli Topping ... 96
35. Hot Tex-Mex Pork Casserole ... 98

BEEF RECIPES ... 100

36. Cauliflower & Beef Casserole ... 100
37. Spiralized Zucchini in Bolognese Sauce ... 102
38. Juicy Beef with Rosemary & Thyme ... 104
39. Red Wine Beef Roast with Vegetables ... 106
40. Grilled Steak with Green Beans ... 108

SEAFOOD RECIPES 110
- 41. COCONUT CRAB PATTIES 110
- 42. SHRIMP IN CURRY SAUCE 112

SMOOTHIES 114
- 43. BERRY BANANA WITH QUINOA SMOOTHIE 114
- 44. VEGAN SANDWICH WITH TOFU & LETTUCE SLAW 115
- 45. GRILLED CAULIFLOWER STEAKS WITH HARICOTS VERT 118
- 46. TOFU & VEGETABLE STIR-FRY 120

SWEETS & DESSERTS RECIPES 122
- 47. CHOCOLATE CANDIES WITH BLUEBERRIES 122
- 48. MATCHA BROWNIES WITH MACADAMIA NUTS 124
- 49. MASCARPONE & STRAWBERRY PUDDING 126
- 50. DARK CHOCOLATE BROWNIES 127

CONCLUSION 130

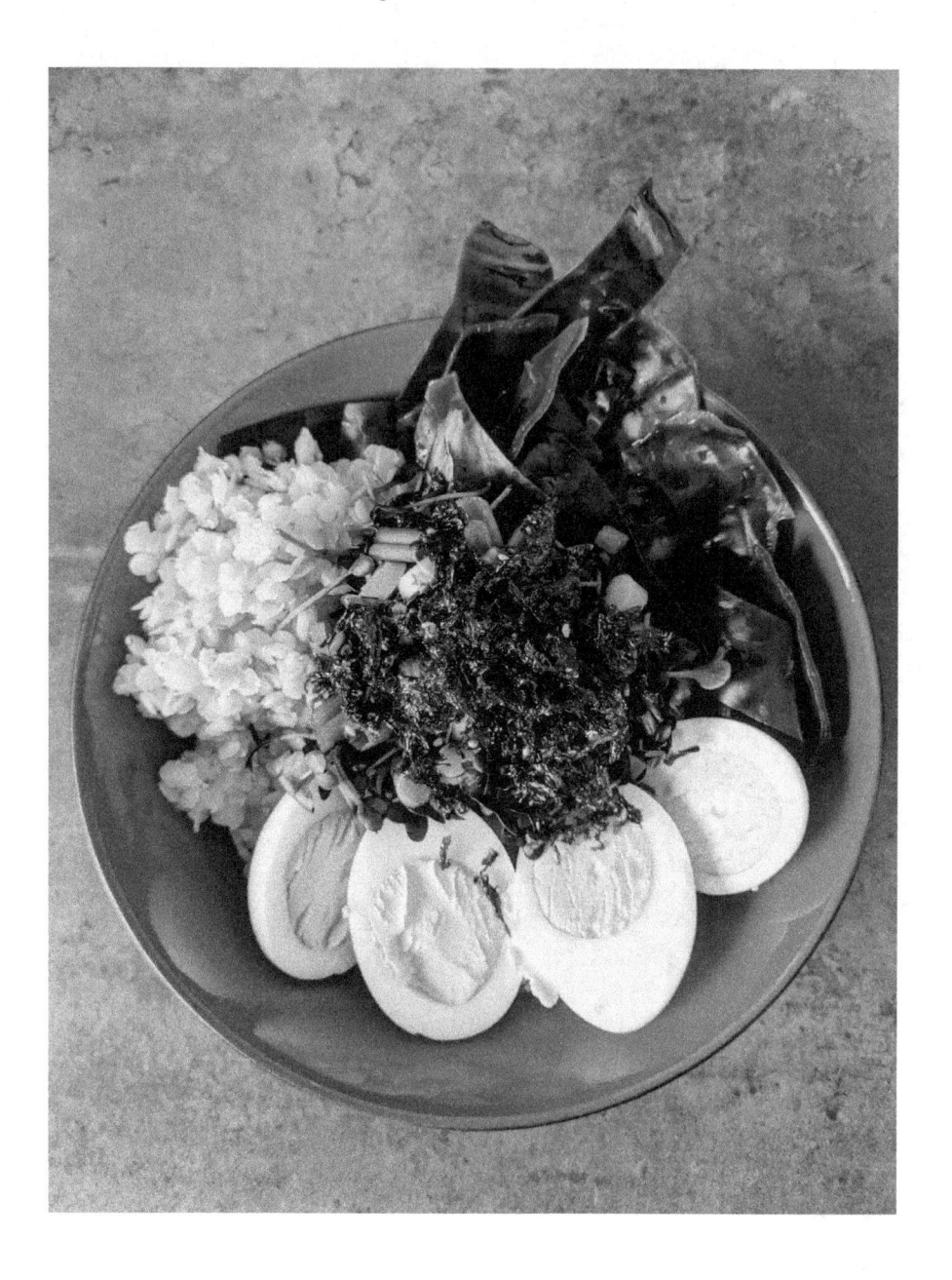

Introduction

When you use a ketogenic diet or lose a lot of weight, your body has to burn through its own fat stores to use as fuel. Over 50 studies show how healthy it is for weight loss, as well as many other health and performance advantages. Because it is recommended by many doctors, it is well-regarded.

As you decrease your carbohydrate intake, you can gain more fat as a greater percentage of your caloric intake is derived from protein on low carb. Being in a low-carb for anaerobic diet causes your body to have a metabolic state known as "ketosis," where fat from your own diet and fat from the rest of your diet is burned for energy.

The ketogenic diet is a quite low-carb, moderate-protein, high-fat diet, which is somewhat similar to the Atkins and the same as the paleo diet

It asks patients to drastically reduce carbohydrate intake and eat lots of fat instead. As you eliminate carbohydrates from your diet, your body enters into a metabolic state called ketosis, or fat metabolism.

When this occurs, your body uses fat as its primary source of energy, your fat oxidation rate skyrockets. When you eat a diet high in carbs, your liver also stores fat. The fat may supply energy for the brain, but if you get enough carbs from the diet to supply your daily needs (6Trusted Source, 7Trusted Source).

The extremely low carbohydrate content of the ketogenic diet may lead to massive reductions in blood sugar and insulin levels. These benefit stretches, such as improved energy, more energy ketones, and decreased inflammation, have many people flocking to the ketogenic diet.

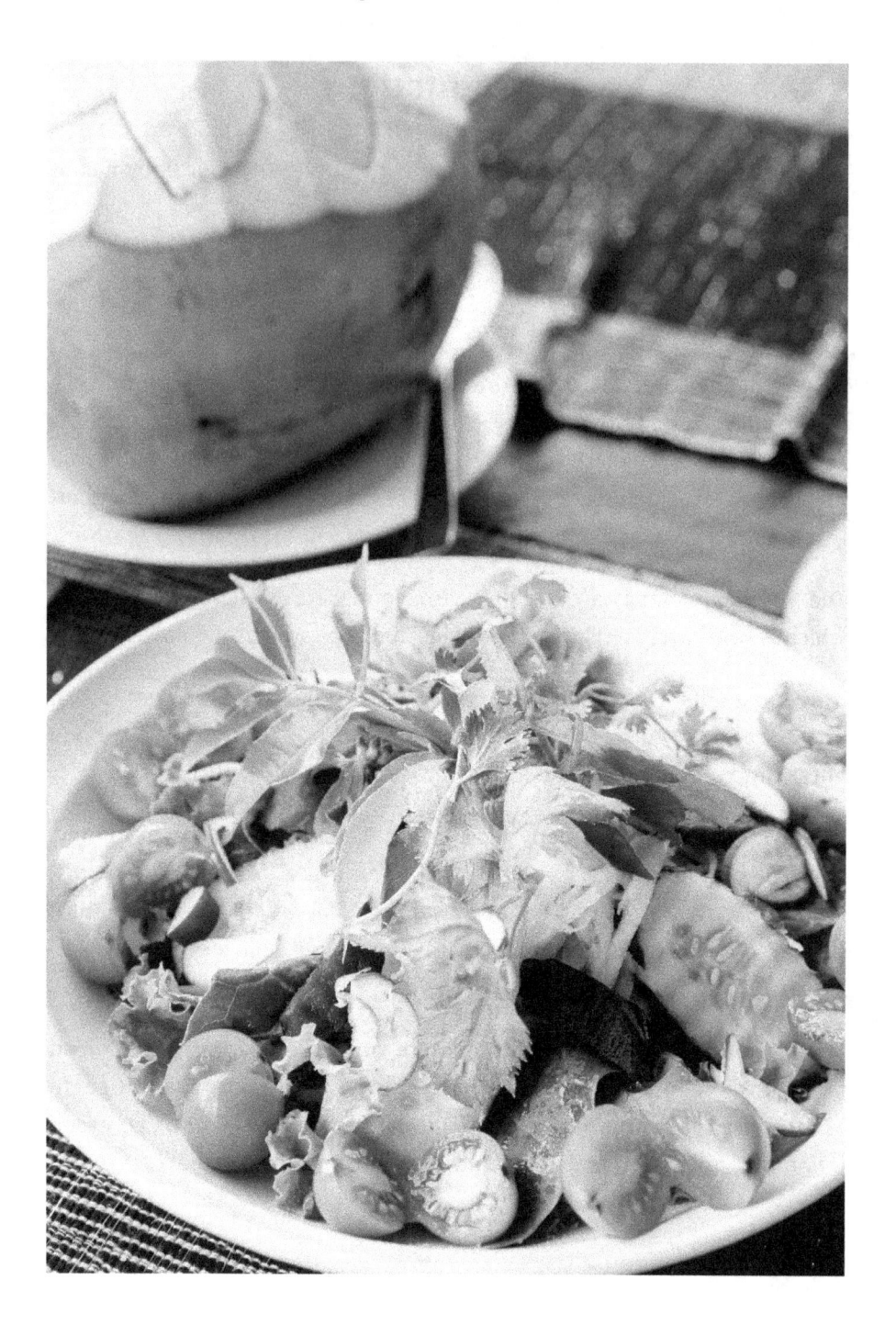

Chapter-1

Is the Ketogenic Diet a Good Choice for Women Over 50?

In their younger adults, calorie expenditure slows by about 50 each day in order to maintain constant body weight.

Reduced exercise, as well as the risk of muscular breakdown and the ability to consume more calories due to a slowdown in metabolism, maybe a difficult to keep off as a constant weight.

A low-carb for women over 50

A few popular weight-loss methods in recent years include a low carbohydrate diet (keto) and fasting, but the keto diet has surged as a popular one recently.

We've received a lot of questions about whether or not following the diet is healthy and if it's doable in the long term.

What is the Ketogenic Diet?

Fasting, which helps the body use fat as a fuel, involves reducing the intake of carbs and increasing fat in the diet, so Keto is a way of increasing the body's fat-burning efficiency.

There is strong evidence to suggest that the ketogenic diet is beneficial for overall health and weight loss.

In particular, ketogenic diets have been successful at improving people's lipid metabolism without exacerbating food cravings that are commonly seen with other diets.

Other research has demonstrated that some people who have type 2 diabetes find that keto is helpful for controlling their symptoms.

That highlights the main principles of the ketogenic diet, which are that (1) fat should be the main source of fuel for the body instead of carbohydrates; (2) carbohydrates should be used as a quick energy source, such as sugar and glycogen stores; and (3) fats have an extremely high calorificaiter utility; and (4) a high calorificatiing diet creates metabolic waste.

The goal of the ketogenic diet is to use ketones for fuel

Lose weight and keep it off with Keto Over 50: An informative guide to implementing the ketogenic diet for women in their 50s

You're using a different fuel during extended periods of exertion, such as when you're exercising or long-distance running, because your body is using fatty acids or ketones instead of sugar.

Producing ketones occurs when you've managed to cut your carb intake and get the right amount of protein while eating a bit more carbs.

When you're eating keto-friendly foods that are digested by your body, your liver helps you to transfer fat into ketones, which can serve as an alternative source of energy for your whole body.

In order to be in ketosis, the body must be using fat as an energy source.

"Expand" is beneficial in some cases in expanding fat breakdown, thus enabling the body to use fat as fuel instead of its usual fuel source and resulting in the breakdown of unwanted fat tissue being more easily gotten rid of.

This method of fat loss not only helps you lose weight, but it helps to stabilize your energy levels and prevent your appetite from decreasing during the day.

The foods that will help you transition into and maintain a state of ketosis are composed of high amounts of omega-3 fatty acids from animal products like salmon, sardines, and herring and low amounts of carbohydrates and protein.

Keto diets work best for women who are over 50 years of age.

When people attempt to eat on the keto diet, it seems a lot more difficult because it's hard to figure out which food has high carbohydrates and which food has low carbohydrates, so it can be incorporated into a lot of people.

Here are a few great foods for women over 50 who are on the keto diet.

The Ultimate Guide to Weight Loss: this book goes beyond the keto basics and helps you put it all together to a keto diet complete food list of everything you should eat for weight loss.

processed meats as the primary source of protein, as well as leaner meats, as they are free of carbs

Fish and seafood, such as fried or breaded fish, are best avoided for the added carbohydrates.

Whether they are fried, poached, boiled, scrambled, or hard-boiled, you can have your eggs however you like; they're prepared.

veget richer, and food: those that grow in the ground gets less

Dairy: Choose dairy products that are high in fat; low-fat options are often sweetened with sugar.

Sources of nuts are good, but it is important to avoid eating too much, especially because they are high in fat

All berries are fine in moderation.

There are a lot of low-carb foods to choose from when following the ketogenic diet, and what you will find here are healthy options in most of the greatest quantity are dairy, meat, fish, cheese, bread, and eggs.

Sugar is the main enemy of insulin target

It's fine to have a little fruit as long as it doesn't add sugar to your diet.

Beers and alcoholic beverages: too many carbohydrates and sugars

The starches in this mix are equal to the number of refined carbohydrates found in white bread, rice, and pasta.

keto-fying your favorite foods

There may be some foods that you dislike that aren't suitable for people who have certain food allergies or sensitivities.

a keto-friendly plate made up of macadamia nuts, plain chicken breast, and unbuttered veggies

Giving yourself the ability to live outside of your comfort zone is always difficult.

Food and recipes have a way of being specific to our families that is difficult to leave behind, whether we want to or not and us.

So, When the type of foods you can't eat change, you can be able to restrict. Fortunately, you can get alternatives to the foods you can't eat, or they'll remain within the limits of keto.

This indicates that you can continue to eat sandwiches and pasta, which in my humble opinion is the best possible combination. This generally applies to a low GI food's long-term benefits: Generally, the best low GI foods should be chosen.

sugar-free bread is 20 times less carb than traditional bread

Not difficult to make, 2-ingreduce recipe

It only needs three ingredients to begin to simmer: rice, water, water, oil, and an open fire.

A cereal low-carb breakfast food

Can women over the age of 50 benefits from the Keto?

One thing you can be sure of with regard to Keto is that there are numerous factors to consider before determining whether or not it is suitable for you; however: It is completely up to you whether or not.

A low-carb for women over 5

As long as you are not afflicted with health problems, a ketogenic diet can be very good for you, especially for weight loss.

The most important thing to bear in mind is to eat a healthy balance of vegetables, proteins, low-fat dairy products, and unprocessed carbohydrates.

Just staying on a diet of whole foods is likely to be the most sustainable because it cuts costs less money and has less environmental impact.

It's important to remember that many studies indicate that attempts to track outcomes of the ketogenic diet aren't reliable. Avoid resorting to an unhealthy means of weight loss, such as fad diets or drastic lifestyle changes, and fasting. Instead, find a healthy eating approach that's good for you.

Just because something hasn't worked in the past doesn't mean it can't work in the future.

A low carbohydrate, high fat, moderate protein, and protein eating plan and diet plan can transform your body.

A ketogenic diet is a high-fat, moderate-protein, adequate-carbohydrate, and low-calorie meal plan, which consists of 75% fat, up to 20% protein, and 5% or fewer carbs in order to keep the protein and carbohydrate consumption within a fairly tight range while having plenty of micronutrients - the micronutrients (vitamins and minerals) needed.

At first, it may seem like you have to be difficult to give up carbohydrates, but it doesn't have to be in order to be done.

You should reduce the number of carbohydrates in your daily meals and snacks while simultaneously increasing the fat and protein content.

The more carbs that are consumed, the less likely the person is to be in a state of ketosis.

Carbs could affect everyone differently; some people may only get into ketosis if they eat at 20 grams per day, but others might require eating more to experience it.

Most people will find it to maintain a low-carbohydrate diet and nutritional ketosis if their carbohydrate intake is under 50% of their total daily calories.

Following a ketogenic diet means sticking to healthy food choices, and avoiding carbohydrate-rich options will lead to long-term weight loss for successful short-term goals.

Ketogenic food to consume

Meals and snacks should be comprised of these items: Fatty meats and higher amounts of vegetables (like avocados, butter, olive oil, olives, and olive oil) and lower amounts of carbohydrates, like bread and higher glycemic vegetables (like broccoli)

If you are concerned about nutritional benefits, you should focus on the production of pastured, organic whole eggs.

Poultry includes both chicken and turkey.

Omega-3 fatty fish: Freshly caught salmon, herring, and mackerel

Red meat: venison, pork, organ meats, and buffalo/bison from grass-fed cattle.

full-fat dairy: butter, full-fat yogurt, and heavy cream

Both red and low-fat, with cream cheese: full-fat cheese, cream cheese, mozzarella, and goat cheese; and goat cheese

These include Macadamia nuts, almonds, walnuts, peanut and sunflower seeds as well as all of these, also pumpkin seeds, ground sunflower seeds, and sesame.

Homemade nut butter, almond, cashew, and coconut butter are all suitable for use in this recipe.

These oils are excellent sources of beneficial fats: coconut oil, olive oil, avocado oil, and canola oil, and avocado oil, and sesame oil

While avocados can be incorporated into almost any dish or into snack food or meal mixtures of your choice

Other vegetables: Broccoli, tomatoes, mushrooms, and peppers (not in their starchy form).

These are commonly known as condiments: salt, pepper, vinegar, lemon juice, fresh herbs, and spices.

foods you should stay away from

A keto diet should not be followed while avoiding carb-rich foods

Some of the following foods should be avoided:

There are a number of different types of bread, baked goods, crackers, dough, and pastries on the menu here, and they're known by different names such as bread, white bread, and dough, as well as whole-wheat rolls.

Bitter things:caffeine: The casein from cow's milk, cocoas, orange juice, and maple sap are all sugar substitutes, but orange juice is more bitter.

Diluted sugar beverages: Soda, fruit juices, syrups, sports drinks, and tea.

Spaghetti, macaroni, and spaghetti.

Grains and other than wheat and rice and oats: Cereals, wheat- and oat-based breakfast foods

Also, starchy vegetables: Potatoes, sweet potatoes, corn, butternut squash, and peas, but these are not your best bets.

Beans and legumes: lentils are good; kidney beans, black beans, chickpeas, lentils are especially excellent.

Fruit: Oranges, pears, pineapples, bananas, and pineapples.

heavy or low-carb or high-carb sauces: barbecue sauce, sugary dressing, and dipping sauces

The list of possible ingredients that may increase a person's weight includes Alcoholic drinks (beer and colas), as well as sugary mixed drinks.

Though carbohydrates should be kept in moderation, low-type fruits such as berries may be consumed in limited amounts as long as you are in ketogenic macros [i.e.e. Carbohydrate-deficient but low in protein and fat].

Processed foods and unhealthy fats (for example, saturated, trans, and hydrogenated fats) can be harmful to your heart.

If you are not interested in meeting certain people or establishing relationships, certain topics or styles of conversation should be avoided:

damaging fats: Margarine, shortenings, and oils that are low in polyunsaturated fats, such as canola and corn oil.

Altered foods such as ready-to-to-eat and fast food, packaged meats, such as hot dogs, and lunch meats and lunch meats.

Artificial colors, preservatives, aspartame, and sweeteners such as sugar are added to these food products to extend their shelf life and make them more aesthetically pleasing, but their chemical components have been shown to lead to many diseases

sugar-free, rice, wheat, soy, and dairy beverages

sugar can be found in a variety of beverages, including juice,;, caffeinated, tea variety of beverages such as iced tea and soft drinks

While on a ketogenic diet, you must avoid high-carb foods just as you would any other carb-rich foods.

So we should cut our sugary beverages like Coke and Pepsi because of the health issues they may cause? It's no small that sugary drinks have been linked to various diseases, like obesity and diabetes?

It is wonderful that there are plenty of tasty, sugar-free diet alternatives for us on the keto diet.

Foods to drink on a low carbohydrate diet might include soft drinks and juices as well as full-fat milk, butter, heavy cream, bacon, and eggs.

WATER: Hydration is fundamental for both adults and children, and you should have it throughout the day.

Excellent soda alternative to carbonated water: Carbonated water has been shown to be a bit acidic and unhealthy; however, carbonated water can be made a lot more sparkly and attractive.

If you want to increase the flavor of your coffee, use heavy cream instead of milk.

Although the unfermented green tea leaves do provide some health benefits, the process of fermentation takes away from the very few that remain, making it not as delicious as unfermented green tea.

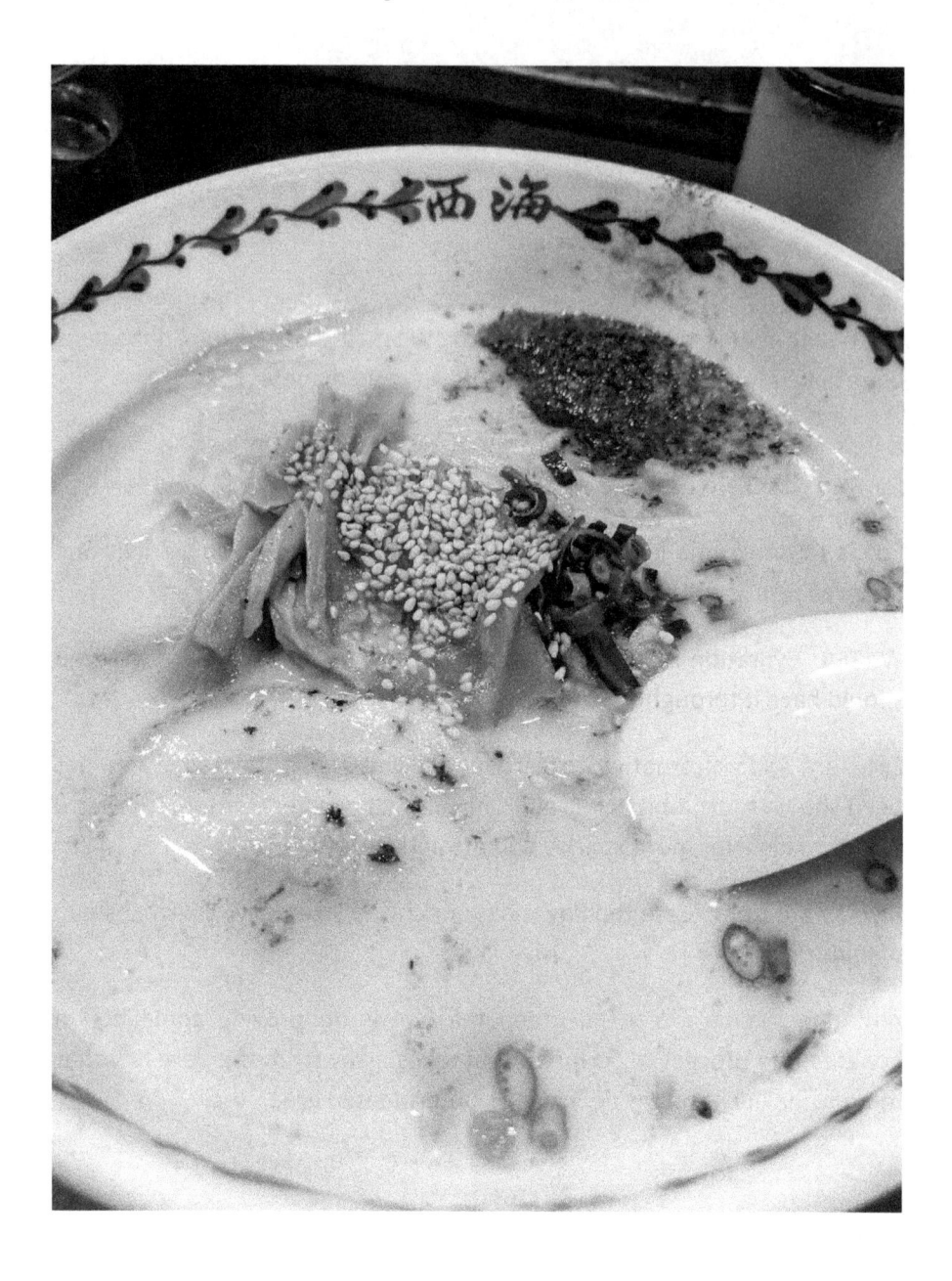

Chapter-2 Over 50 of Our Best Keto Recipes

For many people, new diets represent a new year's resolution. **The ketogenic diet isn't simple (we've been discussing it for several years now), so if you're trying it for the first time, identifying the foods that are right for you is difficult.** As a rule, your choices are usually low carb because that is where your body enters into a state of ketosis or to help your fat burn rather than using carbs for fuel. In order to be able to accomplish this, you must restrict your carbohydrates to about 20 grams of intake. It's not just about cutting carbs, as I like to emphasize; however, the diet is a little more highly adjusted. **P**rocessed foods and sugar are off the table and, and many people no longer eat much or any sweet fruits Alcohol can be enjoyed in moderation. A little dark chocolate can be beneficial, but it's preferable to avoid all dark chocolate as much as possible.

If you'd like to help you understand the potential confusions that arise from following a ketogenic diet, we want to assist you. There are well over 50 recipes in this collection that comply with the requirements of the rule of ketosis, regardless of what you're looking for in them to fit into ketosis. Breakfast through dinner will become a staple for you whether you stay on **a** diet or only for the month.

People who are new to the keto diet might think of bacon and eggs when they envision the typically get started out-of-of-the-the-the-the-box breakfast items, but these can be only the beginning of what you can eat in the morning. Other kinds of fruit, such as smoothies, pancakes, and even whole-grain bread**,** are included.

Return the foods and habits that are outside of the keto diet and lifestyle back into it

a stricter the diet, the fewer micronutrients by-like nutrients that you will be able to get from food. An extended regimen must be necessary to preserve the overall health or for those suffering from adrenal exhaustion or disease.

For the past month, Catherine has been doing a daily multivitamin supplement with Vitamin D and calcium but is now planning to try something different. When you're out working as hard as a mother, you want to ensure you're getting enough nutrients to keep your body running, at the very least. Catherine's daily micronutrients have been covered by her previously named vitamins and minerals.

Micronutrients are depleted by physical activity

A, B, C, magnesium, selenium, manganic acid, potassium, zinc, alpha-lipoic acid, or zinc/selenium, alpha-lipophilic acid

K-friendly diets deprive the body of micronutrients like B vitamins and magnesium

Stress depletes micronutrients such as vitamins, calcium, magnesium, and omega-3 fatty acids deplete both dietary and essential micronutrients.

This is only a partial list of micronutrients that can be used to illustrate the common denominators

We found that frequent training at high levels of training for an extended time both lead to elevated cortisol levels. Do a moderate volume of cycling that is below 75 minutes or a high-intensity cycle that lasts from 45 to 60 minutes to start, and then gradually increase your dosage to maximize cortisol release. a decrease in overall stress levels is critical for a woman who is training for long- or middle-distance running events

And if she gets more rest while training, she will have less stress.

She is tired and reporting problems with her energy levels. When someone is doing an endurance event, this is normal. It is also quite common for women trying to stay on keto after the age of 50 for long periods of time. It is difficult to maintain constant intensity while also listening to your body and enjoying frequent breaks. As a coach, I always want someone below their normal training level. When you're unsure, pause, the cause of fatigue could be either insufficient nutrients or an imbalance of hormones.

Non-nutritive, micronutrients, macronutrients, and macronutrients

her competition targets are reducing inflammation and optimizing her nutrient timing in order to allow her to have energy throughout training and racing. She works out in a very fast and exhausting manner in order to speed herself up the process of recovery for the next time she works out. Maintaining a healthy lean muscular and skeletal composition over the long term is one of her long-term goals.

Catherine might consider which micronutrients to increase because the results of the earlier study seem to indicate she has need of them:

Multivitamin consumed in multiple servings per day

Along with the other key nutrients, such as vitamin B, C, calcium, and Omega 3, appear to play a crucial role in healthy bone growth.

After physical activity, it is necessary to take a good amount of protein nutrition

Nutrition timing after physical activity for most older adults should be between 60 and 120 minutes. One problem: Since Catherine's training is becoming more frequent and intense, her post-exercise smoothie or high protein meal can be met sooner.

To prevent muscle loss, she should aim for 20-35 grams of protein, moderate-based carbohydrate consumption, and keep her carbs low; for reducing inflammation, she should get moderate levels of protein and low to moderate levels of carbs. If certain studies are applied, the findings suggest that older people can obtain similar results to younger people if they have twice the protein intake (40 gm compared to 20).

I like to have all of the ingredients in a blended recovery drink, but I don't always consume it. Including all of the other ingredients are shown to have anti-inflammatory properties

A high-fat, low-carbohydrate, moderate protein, very low-glycemic-index diet

A post-workout smoothie recipe that contains fruit juice and wheat grass-fed gelatin after intense training and cardio

2 quarts spinach2 liters

1/2/2 medium to half an avocado

with about 3/4 cup thawed frozen, pitted, and diced cherries

vegan (dairy-free) paleo and gluten-free, or plant-based protein

a cocoa powder made from cocoa beans (or nibs)

plain, unsweetened coconut milk

Talk to your level of fatigue about how frequently you are feeling it. If your training leaves you feeling fatigued and unable to rest, this may be a sign of overtraining.

A very high-fat, low carbohydrate, moderate protein, moderate-protein, or moderate-high protein diet will help you maintain ketosis while also encourages weight loss of fat.

Above all, whether you are exercising or preparing for a race, you must avoid the risk of developing adrenal fatigue. Following a specific and rigid training program increases the risk of adrenal exhaustion. Do pay attention to the volume of workouts according to your bodily needs; this can ensure that your work/training sessions are not so taxing that you cannot be performed with full strength.

Traditional methods of training for events may stress your body and your body, but giving your body proper nutrition has a high chance of improving your results significantly—or at least minimizing the amount of stress on your body—, is a lot of different.

(progressive) after six months of continual training, I have developed a workout plan that helped keep my cortisol in check and ensured my mass and body composition remained in balance while also enabling me to train progressively. Here is a way to find out about my plans.

Make sure you have a good level of strength training in your routine to prevent injury while also ensures bone retention from increased swimming and biking. They are both great for muscles and bone health, but unlike exercise, they don't provide the bone benefit of weight-bearing.

The best relaxation therapy

Find out how quickly you can go back to regular activities after your illness. If you answer these questions, then you will know how well your nutrition is going to work-outs are going to go. Recovery patterns that persist are typically indicate something long-term. They include constant aches and fatigue or an increase in how hard it is to perform daily activities.

To test your own heart rate, take a quick look in the mirror each morning when you'll Look for the changes in intensity, recovery after extended exercise sessions, rest days, and moderate ones. If your heart rate is consistently increased by 5 BPM over your normal training levels for more than three days, you should take it easy during the remainder of the week and try to get sufficient rest to recuperate and try the following week again.

You can also monitor the variability of the heart rate, which will show a difference between heartbeats.

Let's pretend you have a resting heart rate of 60 beats per minute. You might think that it's just a second long, but it is, in fact, between each beat. This is also an example of the law of diversification in practice: having a wide-ranging selection of heartbeats is ideal. The amount of time could be anywhere between .8 and 1.2 seconds, or perhaps a few smaller. Training may be unpredictable, but rest is not. A more predictable heart rate is better for day-to-to-day gains in aerobic capacity and thus for avoiding burnout.

You need to use special equipment, plus an app, in order to view this content. Both products are consumed first thing in the morning. Use the resting heart rate as a baseline and compare it to a patient's rate before and after treatment.

Finally, one could purchase Sleep Number SleepIQ monitors, which can track your number of hours of sleep per night, allowing one to get a more detailed look at your health and well-being. I prefer it to a device which I can wear. R resting heart rate, HRV, and your sleep duration can help you determine how well you're resting and how you'll benefit from training. A sense of fatigue is important, and finding ways to work around it will help. But if that's a regular occurrence, and if it builds up over time, seek new training balance by doing something else for a while.

Breakfast Recipes

1. Everything Bagel Seasoned Eggs

Macros: Fat: 67% | Protein: 26% | Carbs: 7%

Prep time: 10 minutes | Cook time: 5 minutes | Serves 2

One of the simplest and easiest breakfast of boiled eggs! Spice mixture gives a deliciously spicy kick to boiled eggs.

4 eggs

3 tablespoons white sesame seeds

1 tablespoon black sesame seeds

2 teaspoons poppy seeds

1 tablespoon onion flakes

1 teaspoon garlic flakes

1 teaspoon coarse sea salt

1. In a medium saucepan of water, place the eggs over medium-high heat and bring to a boil. Boil for about 1 minute. Cover the saucepan and immediately remove from the heat. Set the pan aside, covered for about 10 minutes. Drain the eggs and transfer the eggs into a bowl of cold water to cool completely.
2. Meanwhile, in a bowl, mix the remaining ingredients for seasoning.
3. When cooled, peel the eggs and transfer to serving plates. Sprinkle the eggs with some seasoning mixture and serve immediately.

RAGE: Store this seasoning in the sealed jar in the fridge for up to six months.

SERVE IT WITH: Serve these eggs with avocado slices on the side.

PER SERVING

calories: 230 | fat: 17.2g | total carbs: 6.0g | fiber: 2.0g | protein: 14.9g

2. Beef & Veggie Hash

Macros: Fat: 64% | Protein: 27% | Carbs: 9%

Prep time: 15 minutes | Cook time: 35 minutes | Serves 4

One of the best ways to enjoy beef and veggies in your breakfast.

This beef and veggie hash alongside eggs give you a healthy choice to start your day.

2 tablespoons olive oil ½ pound (227 g) ground beef

½ of zucchini, chopped ½ of red bell pepper, seeded and chopped

¼ of onion, chopped 2 teaspoons garlic, minced

1½ cups sugar-free tomato sauce 1 tablespoon dried basil, crushed

1 teaspoon dried oregano, crushed Sea salt and ground black pepper, to taste

4 eggs

1. In a large deep saucepan, heat the oil over medium-high heat and cook the beef for about 10 minutes or until browned, stirring occasionally.

2. Add the zucchini, bell pepper, onion and garlic to cook for about 3 minutes, stirring frequently.

3. Stir in the tomato sauce, dried herbs, salt and black pepper, then bring to a gentle boil. Cook for about 10 minutes, stirring occasionally.

4. With the back of a spoon, make 4 wells in the beef mixture. Carefully, crack 1 egg into each well. Reduce the heat to medium-low and cook covered for about 9 to 10 minutes or until desired doneness.

5. Remove from the heat and serve warm.

STORAGE: Transfer the cooked beef and veggie mixture into a large container and refrigerate for 1 to 2 days.

SERVE IT WITH: Fresh green salad goes great with this dish.

PER SERVING

calories: 268 | fat: 19.2g | total carbs: 8.0g | fiber: 2.0g | protein: 17.8g

3. Eggs & Spinach Florentine

Macros: Fat: 60% | Protein: 36% | Carbs: 4%

Prep time: 10 minutes | Cook time: 5 minutes | Serves 2

A classic egg Florentine that is perfect for an indulgent breakfast!

This classic Eggs Florentine recipe is made with Parmesan spinach with poached eggs.

1 cup fresh spinach leaves, washed completely

2 tablespoons Parmesan cheese, grated freshly

Sea salt and ground black pepper, to taste

1 tablespoon white vinegar

2 eggs

1. In a microwave-safe dish, place the spinach and microwave on High for about 1 to 2 minutes. Remove the bowl from microwave and cut the spinach into bite-sized pieces. Transfer the spinach onto 2 serving plates and sprinkle with Parmesan cheese, salt and black pepper.

2. In a pan of simmering water, add the vinegar and with a spoon, stir quickly. Carefully, break an egg into the center of simmering water. Turn off the heat and cover the pan until the egg is set. Repeat with the remaining egg.

3. Top each plate of spinach with 1 egg and serve.

STORAGE: Transfer the steamed spinach in a container and store in the refrigerator for 1 to 2 days.

REHEAT: Reheat the spinach in microwave and top with poached eggs before serving.

SERVE IT WITH: Serve it with bacon slices.

PER SERVING

calories: 87 | fat: 5.8g | total carbs: 1.1g | fiber: 0.3g | protein: 7.9g

4. Walnut Granola

Macros: Fat 84% | Protein 11% | Carbs 5%

Prep time: 10 minutes | Cook time: 1 hour | Serves 8

The nut granola is a versatile meal. The addition of nuts makes it a nutritious keto diet. You can omit or add other ingredients to suit your preference.

1 cup raw sunflower seeds

2 cups shredded coconut, unsweetened

½ cup walnuts

1 cup almonds, sliced

½ cup raw pumpkin seeds

½ teaspoon nutmeg, ground

10 drops liquid stevia

½ cup coconut oil, melted

1 teaspoon cinnamon, ground

1. Preheat the oven to 250°F (120ºC) and line two baking sheets with parchment paper.
2. In a bowl, add the sunflower seeds, shredded coconut, walnuts, almonds, and pumpkin seeds. Toss well to mix.
3. Add the nutmeg, stevia, coconut oil, and cinnamon in a small bowl, and stir thoroughly to blend.
4. Make the granola mixture: Pour the nutmeg mixture into the sunflower seed mixture and blend well to coat the nuts.
5. Spread the granola mixture on the baking sheets. Arrange the sheets in the preheated oven.
6. Bake for 1 hour or until the granola is crispy and lightly browned. Stir the granola every 15 minutes to break the large pieces.
7. Transfer to serving bowls to cool for 8 minutes before serving.

STORAGE: Store in an airtight container in the fridge for up to 4 days or in the freezer for up to 1 month.

REHEAT: Microwave, covered, until it reaches the desired temperature.

SERVE IT WITH: To make this a complete meal, serve with a cup of unsweetened coffee.

PER SERVING

calories: 397 | fat: 37.0g | total carbs: 10.0g | fiber: 5.0g | protein: 11.0g

5. Creamy Bacon Omelet

Macros: Fat 81% | Protein 15% | Carbs 4%

Prep time: 10 minutes | Cook time: 10 minutes | Serves 4

The meal is easy to prepare and takes a short time to cook. The bacon and pepper add taste and flavor to the meal. You should definitely try out this recipe.

6 eggs

8 cooked and chopped bacon slices

2 tablespoons heavy whipping cream

1 tablespoon olive oil ¼ cup onion, chopped

½ cup canned artichoke hearts, chopped

Sea salt and ground black pepper, to taste

1. In a bowl, whisk the eggs. Add the bacon and cream, then mix well to blend.
2. Heat the olive oil in a skillet over medium-high heat.

3. Sauté the onion in the skillet for 3 minutes or until tender.

4. Make the omelet: Pour the egg mixture into the skillet and swirl the pan so the mixture covers the bottom evenly.

5. Cook the omelet for about 2 minutes. Lift the edges with a spatula to allow the uncooked egg below spread.

6. Sprinkle the artichoke on the omelet, then flip. Cook for an additional 4 minutes or until the omelet becomes firm. Flip again to keep the artichoke on top. Sprinkle salt and pepper to season.

7. Transfer to serving plates to cool before serving.

STORAGE: Store in an airtight container in the fridge for up to 4 days or in the freezer for up to 1 month.

REHEAT: Microwave, covered, until it reaches the desired temperature.

SERVE IT WITH: To make this a complete meal, serve with a light salad.

PER SERVING

calories: 422 | fat: 38.0g | total carbs: 6.0g | fiber: 2.0g | protein: 16.0g

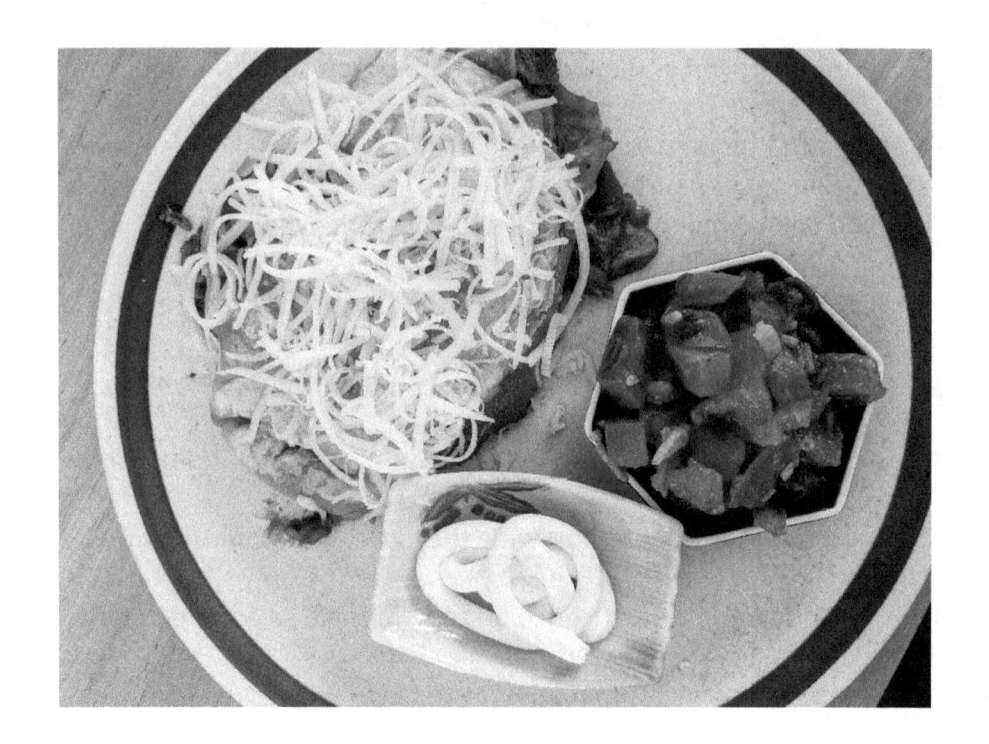

Appetizers and Snacks

6. Tomatoes and Jalapeño Salsa

Macros: Fat 8% | Protein 11% | Carbs 81%

Prep time: 10 minutes | Cook time: 0 minutes | Serves 4

It is an easy to make a recipe that takes only 10 minutes to prepare. The ingredients you use are fresh with lots of nutrients. Best when served immediately after preparation.

4 chopped large tomatoes

½ cup chopped fresh cilantro

1 chopped onion

3 cloves minced garlic

1 diced tomatillo

Salt, to taste

1 tablespoon lime juice

1 minced jalapeño pepper

1. Using a bowl, mix the tomatoes, cilantro, onion, garlic, tomatillo, salt, lime juice and jalapeño pepper. Stir to incorporate.
2. Cover the salsa with plastic wrap. Allow to chill until ready to serve or up to 24 hours.

STORAGE: Store in an airtight container in the fridge for up to 4 days. It is not recommended to freeze.

SERVE IT WITH: To make this a complete meal, serve the dish with zucchini chips.

PER SERVING

calories: 56 | fat: 0.5g | total carbs: 12.3g | fiber: 3.1g | protein: 2.4g

7. Buttered Lobster and Cream Cheese Dip

Macros: Fat 83% | Protein 15% | Carbs 2%

Prep time: 10 minutes | Cook time: 0 minutes | Serves 16

A delicious meal that is suitable when you prepare it a day before eating it. It is creamy and sweet to the taste buds. Why not try this simple recipe?

1 (7-ounce / 198-g) can drained and flaked lobster meat

1 tablespoon lemon juice

1 tablespoon minced onion

4 tablespoons softened butter

1 (8-ounce / 227-g) package softened cream cheese

Salt and freshly ground black pepper, to taste

1. In a bowl, add the lobster meat, lemon juice, onion, butter, cream cheese, pepper, and salt. Mix well until the mixture is smooth.

2. Cover the mixture with plastic wrap, then transfer to the refrigerator and chill until ready to serve.

STORAGE: Store in an airtight container in the fridge for up to 4 days.

SERVE IT WITH: To make this a complete meal, serve it with Bacon Cauliflower Chowder.

PER SERVING

calories: 85 | fat: 7.8g | total carbs: 0.7g | fiber: 0g | protein: 3.0g

8. Prosciutto and Asparagus Wraps

Macros: Fat 21% | Protein 51% | Carbs 28%

Prep time: 15 minutes | Cook time: 15 minutes | Serves 4

It is a special and easy to make a meal. It is suitable for Mother's Day, Easter or any special occasion. When served, the meal is fancy and appealing to the eyes. The salty flavor complements the sweet asparagus flavor.

½ pound (227 g) sliced prosciutto

½ (8-ounce / 227-g) package softened Parmesan cheese

12 spears trimmed fresh asparagus

1. Preheat the oven to 450ºF (235ºC).
2. On a flat work surface, spread the prosciutto slices with the cheese. Tightly wrap the slices around 3 asparagus spears. Repeat with the remaining slices and asparagus spears.
3. Arrange the wrapped spears on a greased baking sheet in a single layer.

4. Transfer to the oven and bake for about 15 minutes until the asparagus spears become tender.

5. Transfer to four serving plates and cool for a few minutes before serving.

STORAGE: Store in an airtight container in the fridge for up to 4 days.

REHEAT: Microwave the sliced prosciutto, covered, until it reaches the desired temperature.

SERVE IT WITH: To make this a complete meal, serve the dish with Creamy Broccoli Cheddar Soup.

PER SERVING

calories: 178 | fat: 4.3g | total carbs: 12.6g | fiber: 0.2g | protein: 22.1g

9. Low-Carb Cheesy Almond Biscuits

Macros: Fat 72% | Protein 25% | Carbs 3%

Prep time: 20 minutes | Cook time: 20 minutes | Serves 8

The biscuits are delicious. For cheese lovers, you won't miss out your favorite cheese. It can make individual biscuits or a large loaf. The biscuits are perfect for both keto and non-keto diet individuals.

1 tablespoon baking powder

2 cups almond flour

2½ cups shredded Cheddar cheese

4 eggs

⅛ cup heavy cream

1. Preheat the oven to 350ºF (180ºC) and line a baking sheet with parchment paper. Set aside.
2. In a bowl, add the baking powder, almond flour and Cheddar cheese. Stir well to mix. In a separate bowl, whisk the eggs until frothy.

3. Make a well in the center of the almond mixture bowl, then gently pour in the whisked eggs and heavy cream. Using a fork, stir the mixture until it forms a sticky batter.

4. Make the biscuits: Divide the batter into 9 equal portions and transfer to the baking sheet, then form into a rounded biscuit shape. Bake for 20 minutes until a toothpick inserted in the center comes out clean.

5. Divide the biscuits among serving plates and allow to cool for 5 minutes before serving.

STORAGE: Store in an airtight container in the fridge for up to 4 days.

REHEAT: Microwave, covered, until it reaches the desired temperature.

SERVE IT WITH: To make this a complete meal, serve the biscuits with a cup of coffee.

PER SERVING

calories: 243 | fat: 19.7g | total carbs: 2.1g | fiber: 0.1g | protein: 14.5g

Dinner Recipes

10. Jamon & Queso Balls

Preparation Time **: 10 minutes**

Cooking Time :30 minutes

Servings **: 6**

Ingredients

- 1 egg
- 6 slices jamon serrano, chopped
- 6 ounces cotija cheese
- 6 ounces Manchego cheese
- Salt and black pepper, to taste
- ¼ cup almond flour 1 tsp baking powder
- **1 tsp garlic powder**

Directions

1. Preheat oven to 420 ºF.

2. Whisk the egg; place in the remaining ingredients and mix well. Split the mixture into 16 balls;

3. Set the balls on a baking sheet lined with parchment paper.

11. Bake for 13 minutes or until they turn golden brown and become crispy.

Nutrition:

- Calories 185

- Total Fats 8.5g

- Carbs: 0g

- Protein 27g

- Dietary Fiber: 0g

12. Cajun Crabmeat Frittata

Preparation Time **: 10 minutes**

Cooking Time: **20 minutes**

Servings **: 6**

Ingredients

- 1 tbsp olive oil
- 1 onion, chopped
- 4 ounces crabmeat, chopped
- 1 tsp cajun seasoning
- 6 large eggs, slightly beaten
- **½ cup Greek yogurt**

Directions

1. Preheat oven to 350ºF. Set a large skillet over medium heat and warm the oil. Add in onion and sauté until soft, about 3 minutes.

2. Stir in crabmeat and cook for 2 more minutes. Season with Cajun seasoning. Evenly distribute the ingredients at the bottom of the skillet.

3. **Whisk the eggs with yogurt. Transfer to the skillet. Set the skillet in the oven and bake for about 18 minutes or until eggs are cooked through. Slice into wedges and serve warm.**

Nutrition :

- Calories 280
- Total Fats 17g
- Carbs: 3g
- Protein 35g
- Dietary Fiber: 1g

13. Crabmeat & Cheese Stuffed Avocado

Preparation Time: **10 minutes**

Cooking Time :50 minutes

Servings **: 6**

Ingredients

- 1 tsp olive oil
- 1 cup crabmeat
- 2 avocados, halved and pitted
- 3 ounces cream cheese
- ¼ cup almonds, chopped
- 1 tsp smoked paprika

Directions

1. Preheat oven to 425ºF and grease a baking pan with cooking spray.

2. In a bowl, mix crabmeat with cream cheese. To the avocado halves, place in almonds and crabmeat/cheese mixture and bake for 18 minutes.

3. Decorate with smoked paprika and serve.

Nutrition: Calories 300 - Total Fats 8g - Carbs: 5g - Protein 18g - Dietary Fiber: 2g

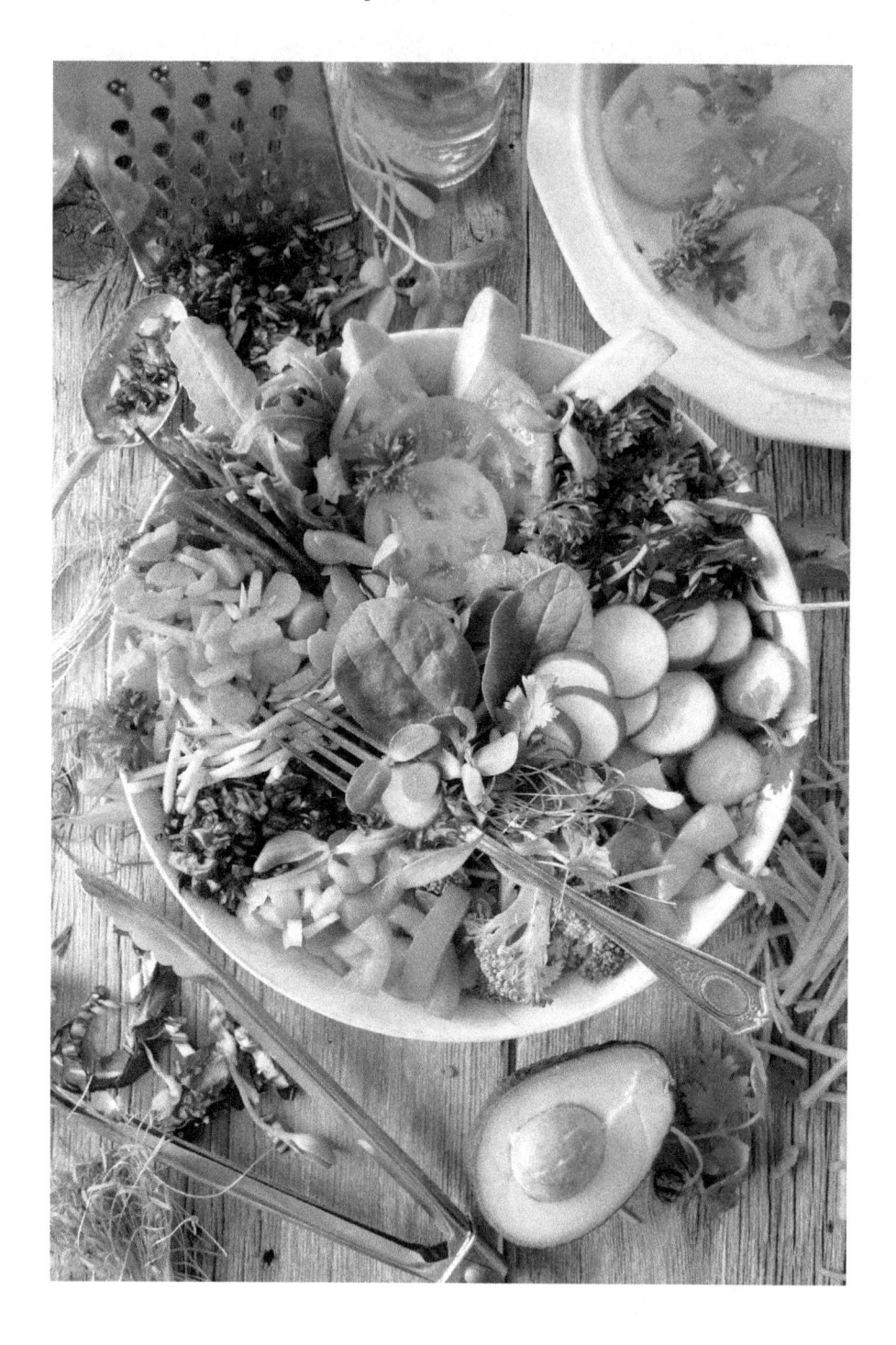

Easy Peasy Recipes

14. Cheesy Brussels Sprouts Salad

Ingredients for 6 servings

2 lb Brussels sprouts, halved

3 tbsp olive oil

Salt and black pepper to taste

2 ½ tbsp balsamic vinegar

¼ red cabbage, shredded

1 tbsp Dijon mustard

1 cup Parmesan, grated

2 tbsp pumpkin seeds, toasted

Instructions - Total Time: around 35 minutes

- Preheat oven to 400 F. Line a baking sheet with foil. Toss brussels sprouts with olive oil, salt, pepper, and balsamic vinegar in a bowl and spread on the baking sheet.
- Bake for 20-25 minutes. Transfer to a salad bowl and mix in red cabbage, mustard, and half of the cheese.

- Sprinkle with the remaining cheese and pumpkin seeds and serve.

Per serving: Cal 210; Net Carbs 6g; Fat 18g; Protein 4g

15. Tomato Bites with Vegan Cheese Topping

Ingredients for 4 servings

2 spring onions, chopped

5 tomatoes, sliced

¼ cup olive oil

1 tbsp seasoning mix

For vegan cheese

½ cup pepitas seeds

1 tbsp nutritional yeast

Salt and black pepper, to taste

1 tsp garlic puree

Instructions - Total Time: around 15 minutes

Drizzle tomatoes with olive oil. Preheat oven to 400 F. In a food processor, add all vegan cheese ingredients and pulse until the desired consistency is attained. Combine vegan cheese and seasoning mix. Toss in the tomato slices to coat. Set tomato slices on a baking pan and bake for 10

minutes. Top with spring onions and serve.

Per serving: Cal 161; Net Carbs: 7g; Fat: 14g; Protein: 5g

16. Salami Cauliflower Pizza

Ingredients for 4 servings

2 cups grated mozzarella

¼ cup tomato sauce

4 cups cauliflower rice

4 oz salami slices

1 tbsp dried thyme

Instructions - Total Time: around 40 minutes

Preheat oven to 390 F. Microwave cauliflower rice mixed with 1 tbsp of water for 1 minute. Remove and mix in 1 cup of the mozzarella cheese and thyme. Pour the mixture into a greased baking dish, spread out and bake for 5 minutes. Remove the dish and spread the tomato sauce on top. Scatter remaining mozzarella cheese on the sauce and then arrange salami slices on top. Bake for 15 minutes.

Per serving: Cal 276; Net Carbs 2g; Fats 15g; Protein 20g

17. Baked Cheese & Cauliflower

Ingredients for 4 servings

1 head cauliflower, cut into florets

¼ cup butter, cubed

2 tbsp melted butter

1 white onion, chopped

¼ almond milk

½ cup almond flour

1 ½ cups grated Colby cheese

Instructions - Total Time: around 30 minutes

Preheat oven to 350 F. Microwave the cauli florets for 4-5 minutes. Melt the butter cubes in a saucepan and sauté onion for 3 minutes. Add in cauliflower, season with salt and pepper, and mix in almond milk. Simmer for 3 minutes. Mix the remaining melted butter with almond flour. Stir into the cauliflower as well as half of the cheese. Sprinkle the top with the remaining cheese and bake for 10 minutes. Plate the bake and serve with arugula salad.

Per serving: Cal 215; Net Carbs 4g; Fat 15g; Protein 12g

18. Spanish Paella "Keto-Style"

Ingredients for 4 servings

½ pound rabbit, cut into pieces

½ pound chicken drumsticks

1 white onion, chopped

2 garlic cloves, minced

1 red bell pepper, chopped

2 tbsp olive oil

½ cup thyme, chopped

1 tsp smoked paprika

2 tbsp tomato puree

½ cup white wine

1 cup chicken broth

2 cups cauli rice

1 cup green beans, chopped

A pinch of saffron

Instructions - Total Time: around 70 minutes

Preheat oven to 350 F. Warm olive oil in a pan. Fry chicken and rabbit on all sides for 8 minutes; remove to a plate. Add onion and garlic to the pan and sauté for 3 minutes. Include in tomato puree, bell pepper, and smoked paprika and let simmer for 2 minutes.

Pour in broth and simmer for 6 minutes. Stir in cauli rice, white wine, green beans, saffron, and thyme and lay the meat on top. Transfer the pan to the oven and cook for 20 minutes. Season and serve.

Per serving: Cal 378; Net Carbs 7.6g; Fat 21g; Protein 37g

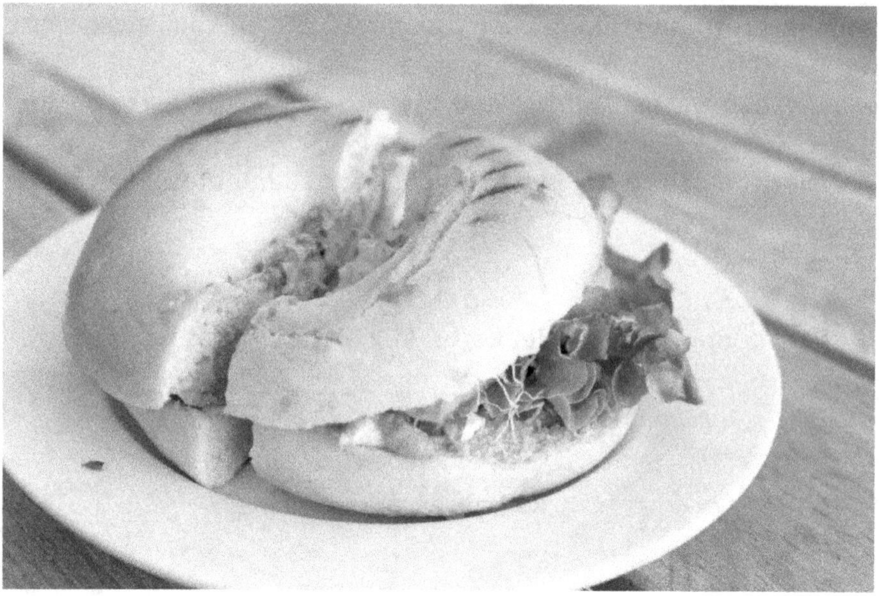

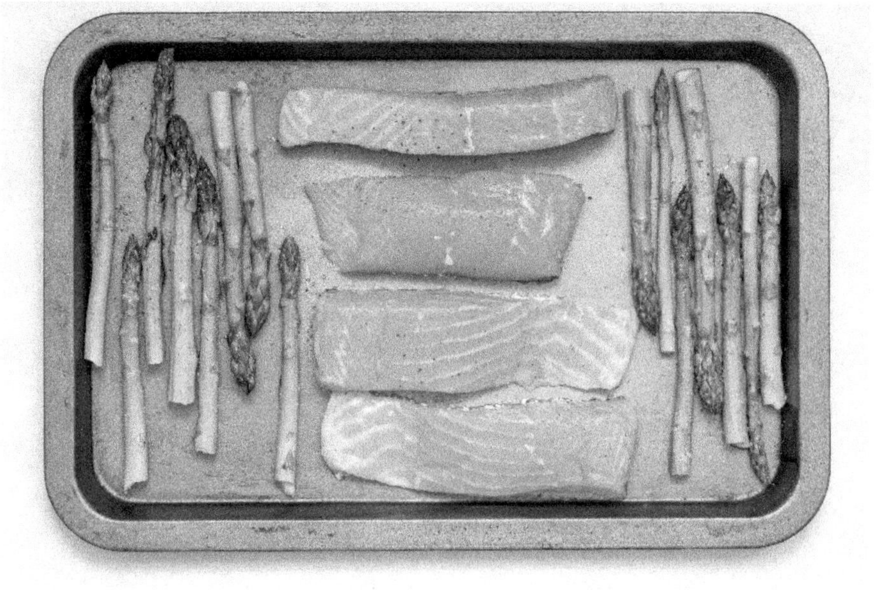

Salads & Soups Recipes

19. Modern Greek Salad with Avocado

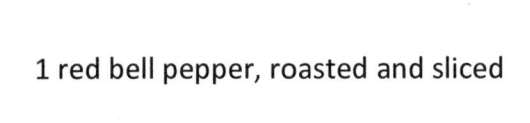

Ingredients **for 2 servings**

1 red bell pepper, roasted and sliced

2 tomatoes, sliced

1 avocado, sliced

6 kalamata olives

¼ lb feta cheese, sliced

1 tbsp vinegar

1 tbsp olive oil

1 tbsp parsley, chopped

Directions **and Total Time: approx. 10 minutes**

Arrange the tomato slices on a serving platter and place the avocado slices in the middle. Place the olives and bell pepper around the avocado slices and drop pieces of feta on the platter. Drizzle with olive oil and vinegar and sprinkle with parsley to serve.

Per serving: Cal 411; Fat 35g; Net Carbs 5.2g; Protein 13g

20. Seared Rump Steak Salad

Ingredients **for 2 servings**

1 cup green beans, steamed and sliced

½ lb rump steak

3 green onions, sliced

3 tomatoes, sliced

1 avocado, sliced

2 cups Romaine lettuce, torn

2 tsp yellow mustard

Salt and black pepper to taste

3 tbsp extra virgin olive oil

1 tbsp balsamic vinegar

Directions and Total Time: approx. 20 minutes

In a bowl, mix the mustard, salt, black pepper, balsamic vinegar, and extra virgin olive oil. Set aside.

Preheat a grill pan over high heat while you season the meat with salt and pepper. Place the steak in the pan and brown for 4 minutes per side. Remove to a chopping board and let it sit for 4 minutes before slicing.

In a salad bowl, add the green onions, tomatoes, green beans, lettuce, and steak slices. Drizzle the dressing over and toss to coat. Top with avocado slices and serve.

Per serving: Cal 611; Fat 45g; Net Carbs 6.4g; Protein 33g

21. Cheesy Beef Salad

Ingredients for 4 servings

½ lb beef rump steak, cut into strips

1 tsp cumin

3 tbsp olive oil

Salt and black pepper to taste

1 tbsp thyme

1 garlic clove, minced

½ cup ricotta, crumbled ½ cup pecans, toasted

2 cups baby spinach 1 ½ tbsp lemon juice

¼ cup fresh mint, chopped

Directions and Total Time: approx. 15 minutes

Preheat the grill to medium heat. Rub the beef with salt, 1 tbsp of olive oil, garlic, thyme, black pepper, and cumin. Place on the preheated grill and cook for 10 minutes, flipping once.

Sprinkle the pecans on a dry pan over medium heat and cook for 2-3 minutes, shaking frequently. Remove the grilled beef to a cutting board, leave to cool, and slice into strips. In a salad bowl, combine baby spinach with mint, remaining olive oil, salt, lemon juice, ricotta, and pecans, and toss well to coat. Top with the beef slices.

Per serving: Cal 437; Fat 42g; Net Carbs 4.2g; Protein 16g

22. Pickled Pepper Salad with Grilled Stea k

Ingredients **for 2 servings**

½ cup feta cheese, crumbled

1 lb skirt steak, sliced

Salt and black pepper to taste

1 tsp olive oil

1 cup lettuce salad

1 cup arugula

3 pickled peppers, chopped

2 tbsp red wine vinegar

Directions **and Total Time: approx. 15 minutes**

Preheat grill to high heat. Season the steak slices with salt and black pepper and drizzle with olive oil. Grill the steaks on each side to the desired doneness, about 5-6 minutes. Remove to a bowl, cover, and leave to rest while you make the salad. Mix the lettuce salad and arugula, pickled peppers, and vinegar in a salad bowl. Add the beef and sprinkle with feta cheese.

Per serving: Cal 633; Fat 34g; Net Carbs 4.7g; Protein 72g

23. Parma Ham & Egg Salad

Ingredients **for 4 servings**

8 eggs

1/3 cup mayonnaise

1 tbsp minced onion

½ tsp mustard

1 ½ tsp lime juice

Salt and black pepper, to taste

10 lettuce leaves

4 Parma ham slices

Directions **and Total Time: approx. 20 minutes**

Boil the eggs for 10 minutes in a pot filled with salted water. Remove and run under cold water. Then peel and chop. Transfer to a mixing bowl together with the mayonnaise, mustard, black pepper, lime juice, onion, and salt. Top with lettuce leaves and ham slices to serve.

Per serving: Cal 723; Fat 53g; Net Carbs 5.6g; Protein 47g

24. Chicken Salad with Gorgonzola Cheese

Ingredients for 2 servings

½ cup gorgonzola cheese, crumbled

1 chicken breast, boneless, skinless, flattened

Salt and black pepper to taste

1 tbsp garlic powder

2 tsp olive oil

1 cup arugula

1 tbsp red wine vinegar

Directions and Total Time: approx. 15 minutes

Rub the chicken with salt, black pepper, and garlic powder. Heat half of the olive oil in a pan over medium heat and fry the chicken for 4 minutes on both sides or until golden brown. Remove to a cutting board and let cool before slicing.

Toss the arugula with vinegar and the remaining olive oil; share the salads onto plates. Arrange the chicken slices on top and sprinkle with gorgonzola cheese.

Per serving: Cal 291; Fat 24g; Net Carbs 3.5g; Protein 12g

Poultry Recipes

25. Spicy Garlic Chicken Kebabs

Macros: Fat: 50% | Protein: 44% | Carbs: 6%

Prep time: 15 minutes | Cook time: 12 minutes | Serves 6

C hicken kebabs has always been a party pleaser but this spicy variation will kick your party up a notch. It can be stored and reheated which makes it a suitable leftover meal and can replace carb-laden snacks.

1 cup plain Greek yogurt

2 tablespoons freshly squeezed lemon juice, or more to taste

1 tablespoon kosher salt

1½ teaspoons ground cumin

1 teaspoon freshly ground black pepper

⅛ teaspoon ground cinnamon

2 tablespoons olive oil, divided

6 cloves garlic, minced

1 tablespoon red pepper flakes

1 teaspoon paprika

2½ pounds (1.1 kg) boneless, skinless chicken thighs, halved

SPECIAL EQUIPMENT:

4 long metal skewers

1. Mix the yogurt, lemon juice, kosher salt, cumin, black pepper, cinnamon, 1 tablespoon olive oil, garlic, red pepper flakes, and paprika together in a bowl.
2. Put the chicken in the marinade to coat, then cover the bowl with plastic wrap and refrigerate to marinate for 2 to 8 hours.
3. Preheat the grill to medium-high heat and brush the grill grates with the remaining olive oil.
4. Make the kebabs: Thread half of the chicken on two skewers and shape it into a thick log.
5. Put the kebabs on the grill and cook for 4 to 5 minutes. Flip the kebabs over and cook the for about 6 minutes more, or until

cooked through and a meat thermometer inserted in the center registers 165ºF (74ºC).

6. Remove the kebabs from the grill and serve on a plate.

STORAGE: Store in an airtight container in the fridge for up to 4 days or in the freezer for up to 1 month.

REHEAT: Microwave, covered, until the desired temperature is reached or reheat in a frying pan or air fryer / instant pot, covered, on medium.

SERVE IT WITH: To make this a complete meal, serve it with a bowl of green salad.

PER SERVING

calories: 512 | fat: 28.5g | total carbs: 11.7g | fiber: 4.1g | protein: 56.3g

26. Cheesy Chicken Dish With Spinach

Macros: Fat: 54% | Protein: 40% | Carbs: 6%

Prep time: 10 minutes | Cook time: 15 minutes | Serves 4

This mouth-watering cheesy chicken dish with spinach and tomatoes is just bursting with flavorful deliciousness. It is a family favorite dish and can bring any boring dish to life. Dip your fork into this cheesy deliciousness and you certainly won't regret it.

2 tablespoons olive oil   ½ pounds (680 g) skinless, boneless chicken breast, thinly sliced   1 cup heavy cream   1 teaspoon garlic powder

1 teaspoon Italian seasoning   ½ cup chicken broth

½ cup Parmesan cheese, grated   1 cup spinach, chopped

½ cup sun-dried tomatoes, chopped

1. Heat the olive oil in a large skillet over medium-high heat.
2. Add the chicken to the skillet and cook for 3 to 5 minutes on each side or until lightly browned. Transfer the chicken to a plate and set aside.

3. Pour the heavy cream in the skillet and add the garlic powder, Italian seasoning, chicken broth, and Parmesan cheese, then whisk well for 5 minutes or until the sauce starts to thicken.

4. Mix in the spinach and the tomatoes and cook on low heat for 1 minute. Put the chicken back into the skillet and cook for 2 to 3 minutes. Keep stirring during the cooking.

5. Remove from the heat and serve on plates.

STORAGE: Store in an airtight container in the fridge for up to 4 days or in the freezer for up to 1 month.

REHEAT: Microwave, covered, until the desired temperature is reached or reheat in a frying pan or instant pot, covered, on medium.

SERVE IT WITH: To make this a complete meal, serve it with Greek salad or coleslaw.

PER SERVING

calories: 437 | fat: 26.1g | total carbs: 7.7g | fiber: 1.2g | protein: 44.0g

27. Delicious Parmesan Chicken

Macros: Fat 75% | Protein 23% | Carbs 2%

Prep time: 20 minutes | Cook time: 8 minutes | Serves 4

The kids will enjoy this delicious Parmesan chicken especially for dinner. The chicken is enriched with essential nutrients from the cream, pork rinds, eggs, and Parmesan cheese. It is a fulfilling recipe for keto diet.

1 (8-ounce / 227-g) skinless, boneless chicken breast

1 tablespoon heavy whipping cream

1 egg

½ teaspoon salt

½ teaspoon red pepper flakes

1 ounce (28 g) grated Parmesan cheese

1½ ounces (43 g) crushed pork rinds

½ teaspoon ground black pepper

½ teaspoon garlic powder

½ teaspoon Italian seasoning

1 tablespoon butter

¼ cup shredded Mozzarella cheese

1. Start by preheating the oven's broiler and put the oven rack about 6 inches from the heat source.
2. On a flat work surface, slice the chicken breast horizontally through the middle, Pound the chicken to ½-inch thickness with a meat mallet.
3. In a bowl, beat the cream and the egg until smooth. Set aside.
4. In another bowl, combine the salt, red pepper flakes, Parmesan cheese, pork rinds, black pepper, garlic powder, and Italian seasoning. Transfer the breading mixture to a plate.
5. Dip the chicken into the egg mixture, then press the chicken into the breading mixture to coat thickly on both sides.
6. Melt the butter in a skillet over medium-high heat.
7. Cook the chicken for about 3 minutes per side, or until it is no longer pink and juices are clear.

8. Put the cooked chicken in a baking tray then top up with Mozzarella cheese.

9. Broil in the preheated oven for about 2 minutes until the cheese is barely brown and bubbly.

STORAGE: Store in an airtight container in the fridge for up to 1 week.

REHEAT: Microwave, covered, until the desired temperature is reached or reheat in a frying pan or air fryer, covered, on medium.

SERVE IT WITH: To make this a complete meal, serve the Parmesan chicken with zucchini noodles.

PER SERVING

calories: 492 | fat: 41.2g | total carbs: 2.5g | fiber: 0.4g | protein:28.1g

28. Michigander-Style Turkey

Macros: Fat 40% | Protein 59% | Carbs 1%

Prep time: 10 minutes | Cook time: 4 hours | Serves 16

Wondering what to prepare your entire family for dinner?

Michigander-style turkey will sort out all your worries. During the last minutes of cooking, remember to remove the foil so that the turkey browns nicely. 1 (12-pound / 5.4-kg) whole turkey

6 tablespoons butter, divided 3 tablespoons chicken broth

4 cups warm water 2 tablespoons dried onion, minced

2 tablespoons dried parsley 2 tablespoons seasoning salt

1. Start by preheating the oven to 35 0°F (18 0°C).
2. Rinse the turkey and pat dry with paper towels.
3. Put the turkey on a roasting pan, then separate the skin over the breast to make pockets.
4. Put 3 tablespoons of butter into each pocket.
5. Mix the broth and water in a medium bowl.

6. Add the minced onion and parsley, then pour over the turkey. Sprinkle some salt on the turkey then cover with aluminum foil.
7. Bake in the preheated oven until the internal temperatures of the turkey reads 180°F (8 0°C), for about 4 hours.
8. When 45 minutes are remaining, remove the foil so that the turkey browns well.
9. Remove from the oven and serve warm.

STORAGE: Store in an airtight container in the fridge for up to 1 week

REHEAT: Microwave, covered, until the desired temperature is reached or reheat in an air fryer covered, on medium.

SERVE IT WITH: To make this a complete meal, serve the turkey with sautéed garlic kale and lemon.

PER SERVING

calories: 497 | fat: 22.1g | total carbs: 0.6g | fiber: 0g | protein: 73.8g

29. Keto Chicken Casserole

Macros: Fat 46% | Protein 46% | Carbs 8%

Prep time: 15 minutes | Cook time: 25 minutes | Serves 4

Keto chicken casserole is a recipe you have come across not once but several times. However, it is worth cooking over and over again because of its great taste and essential nutrients especially on keto diet. This recipe is perfect for dinner.

4 skinless, boneless chicken breast halves

¼ cup butter

1 tablespoon Italian seasoning

3 teaspoons minced garlic

½ cup grated Parmesan cheese

1 tablespoon lemon juice

½ cup heavy cream

1 (10 ¾ -ounce / 305-g) can condensed cream of mushroom soup

2 (13 ½ -ounce / 383-g) cans drained spinach

4 ounces (113 g) fresh sliced mushrooms

⅔ cup bacon bits

2 cups shredded Mozzarella cheese

1. Start by preheating the oven to 350 °F (180 °C), then put the chicken breast halves on a greased baking tray.
2. Bake in the preheated oven for 30 minutes until the juices are clear. Remove from the oven and put aside.
3. Increase the temperatures in the oven to 400 °F (205 °C).
4. Melt the butter in a medium saucepan over medium heat.
5. Add the Italian seasoning, garlic, Parmesan cheese, lemon juice, heavy cream, and mushroom soup, stirring continuously, for about 4 minutes. Set aside.
6. Place the spinach at the bottom of a baking dish.
7. Add the mushrooms then pour ½ of the mixture from the saucepan on top.
8. Place the chicken then pour the remaining sauce mixture.
9. Sprinkle the bacon bits then top with Mozzarella cheese.

10. Bake in the preheated oven for about 25 minutes until the chicken is lightly browned and the cheese is bubbly.

11. Remove form the oven and slice to serve.

STORAGE: Store in an airtight container in the fridge for up to 1 week

REHEAT: Microwave, covered, until the desired temperature is reached or reheat in an air fryer, covered, on medium.

SERVE IT WITH: To make this a complete meal, serve the chicken casserole with buttered mushrooms.

PER SERVING

calories: 717 | fat: 36.6g | total carbs: 21.3g | fiber: 6.3g | protein: 81.9g

30. Almond Chicken Cordon Bleu

Macros: Fat 46% | Protein 52% | Carbs 2%

Prep time: 10 minutes | Cook time: 35 minutes | Serves 4

If you want to surprise your family with a unique and tasty chicken recipe, then go for almond chicken cordon bleu. The almond flavor gives the chicken a tasty approach that will leave you craving for more. For best results, use a chicken breast without bones.

2 tablespoons olive oil

4 skinless, boneless chicken breast halves

⅛ teaspoon ground black pepper

¼ teaspoon salt

6 slices Swiss cheese

4 slices cooked ham ½ cup almond meal

SPECIAL EQUIPMENT:

Toothpicks, soaked for at least 30 minutes

1. Start by preheating the oven to 350 °F (180 °C) then grease a baking sheet with olive oil.
2. On a flat work surface, using a meat mallet to pound the chicken until it is ¼-inch thickness.
3. Sprinkle the pepper and salt on each piece of the chicken evenly.
4. Put 1 slice of ham and 1 slice of cheese on each breast.
5. Roll each breast and tightly secure with a toothpick.
6. Arrange them on the prepared baking sheet and evenly sprinkle with the almond meal.
7. Bake in the preheated oven until cooked through, for about 35 minutes
8. Remove from the oven and top each breast with ½ cheese slice.
9. Return to the oven and bake for 5 minutes more, until the cheese is bubbly.
10. Remove from the oven and serve on plates.

STORAGE: Store in an airtight container in the fridge for up to 1 week

REHEAT: Microwave, covered, until the desired temperature is reached or reheat in an air fryer, covered, on medium.

SERVE IT WITH: To make this a complete meal, serve the almond chicken cordon bleu with saucy chili-garlic cucumber noodles

PER SERVING

calories: 532 | fat: 27.1g | total carbs: 3.4g | fiber: 0.4g | protein: 69.1g

Pork Recipes

31. Chorizo in Cabbage Sauce with Pine Nuts

Ingredients for 4 servings

1 head green canon cabbage, shredded

6 tbsp butter

25 oz chorizo sausages

1 ¼ cups coconut cream

½ cup fresh sage, chopped

½ lemon, zested

2 tbsp toasted pine nuts

Instructions - Total Time: around 30 minutes

Melt 2 tbsp of butter in a skillet over medium heat and fry chorizo until lightly brown on the outside, 10 minutes. Remove to a plate. Melt the remaining butter and sauté cabbage, occasionally stirring, 4 minutes. Mix in coconut cream and simmer until the cream reduces by half. Sprinkle with sage and lemon zest. Divide the chorizo into plates, spoon the cabbage to the side of the chorizo, and sprinkle the pine nuts on top. Serve warm.

Per serving: Cal 914; Net Carbs 16g; Fat 76g; Protein 38g

32. Hawaiian Pork Loco Moco

Ingredients for 4 servings

1 ½ lb ground pork

1/3 cup flaxseed meal

1 cup sliced oyster mushrooms

½ tsp nutmeg powder

1 cup vegetable stock

1 tsp onion powder

1 tsp Worcestershire sauce

5 large eggs

1 tsp tamari sauce

2 tbsp heavy cream

½ tsp xanthan gum

3 tbsp coconut oil

2 tbsp olive oil

1 tbsp salted butter

4 large eggs

1 shallot, finely chopped

Instructions - Total Time: around 40 minutes

In a bowl, combine ground pork, flaxseed meal, nutmeg and onion powders. In another bowl, whisk 1 egg with heavy cream and mix into the pork mixture. The batter will be sticky. Mold 8 patties from the mixture; set aside. Heat coconut oil in a skillet over medium heat. Fry the patties on both sides until no longer pink, 8-10 minutes; set aside. Melt the butter in the same skillet and cook shallot and mushrooms until softened, 7 minutes. In a bowl, mix vegetable stock, Worcestershire and tamari sauces. Pour the mixture over the mushrooms and cook for 3 minutes. Stir in xanthan gum and allow thickening, about 1 minute. Heat half of the olive oil in a skillet, crack in an egg, and fry sunshine style, 1 minute. Plate and fry the remaining eggs using the remaining olive oil. Serve pork with mushroom gravy and top with fried eggs.

Per serving: Cal 655; Net Carbs 2.2g; Fat 46g; Protein 55g

33. Pork Sausage Omelet with Mushrooms

Ingredients for 2 servings

1 small white onion, chopped

¼ cup sliced cremini mushrooms

2 tbsp butter

2 tbsp olive oil

6 eggs

2 oz pork sausage, crumbled

2 oz shredded cheddar cheese

Instructions - Total Time: around 30 minutes

- Heat olive oil in a pan over medium heat, add in pork sausage, and fry for 10 minutes; set aside. In the same pan sauté the onion and mushrooms, 8 minutes; set aside.
- Melt the butter over low heat. Beat the eggs into a bowl until smooth and frothy.
- Pour the eggs into the pan, swirl to spread around and omelet begins to firm, top with sausages, mushroom-onion mixture, and cheddar cheese. Using a spatula,

carefully remove the egg mixture around the edges of the pan and flip over the stuffing, and cook for about 2 minutes. Serve warm for breakfast or brunch.

Per serving: Cal 534; Net Carbs 2.7g; Fat 43g; Protein 29g

34. British Pork Pie with Broccoli Topping

Ingredients for 4 servings

1 head broccoli, cut into florets

½ cup crème fraîche

1 whole egg

½ celery, finely chopped

3 oz butter, melted

5 oz shredded Swiss cheese

2 tbsp butter, cold

2 lb ground pork

2 tbsp tamari sauce

2 tbsp Worcestershire sauce

½ tbsp hot sauce

1 tsp onion powder

Instructions - Total Time: around 55 minutes

Preheat oven to 400 F. Bring a pot of salted water to boil and cook broccoli for 3-5 minutes. Drain and transfer to a food processor; grind until rice-like. Transfer to a bowl. Add in crème fraiche, egg, celery, butter, and half of the Swiss cheese. Mix to combine. Melt the cold butter in a pot, add, and cook the pork until brown, 10 minutes. Mix in tamari, hot and Worcestershire sauces, and onion powder; cook for 3 minutes. Spread the mixture on a greased baking dish and cover with broccoli mixture. Sprinkle with the remaining cheese and bake for 20 minutes. Serve.

Per serving: Cal 701; Net Carbs 3.3g; Fat 49g; Protein 60g

35. Hot Tex-Mex Pork Casserole

Ingredients for 4 servings

2 tbsp butter

1 ½ lb ground pork

½ cup shredded Monterey Jack

3 tbsp Tex-Mex seasoning

1 scallion, chopped to garnish

2 tbsp chopped jalapeños

1 cup sour cream, for serving

½ cup crushed tomatoes

Instructions - Total Time: around 40 minutes

- Preheat oven to 330 F. Grease a baking dish with cooking spray. Melt butter in a skillet over medium heat and cook the pork until brown, 8 minutes. Stir in Tex-Mex
- seasoning, jalapeños, and tomatoes; simmer for 5 minutes. Transfer the mixture to the dish and use a spoon to level at the bottom of the dish.

- Sprinkle the Monterey Jack cheese on top and bake for 20 until the cheese melts and is golden brown. Garnish with scallion and sour cream and serve.

Per serving: Cal 431; Net Carbs 7.8g; Fat 24g; Protein 43g

Beef Recipes

36. Cauliflower & Beef Casserole

Ingredients for 4 servings

2 tbsp olive oil

1 lb ground beef

Salt and black pepper to taste

½ cup cauli rice

1 tbsp parsley, chopped

1 cup kohlrabi, chopped

5 oz can diced tomatoes

½ cup mozzarella cheese, grated

Directions and Total Time: approx. 40 minutes

Warm the olive oil in a pot over medium heat. Cook the beef for 5-6 minutes until no longer pink, breaking apart with a wooden spatula. Add cauli rice, kohlrabi, tomatoes, and ¼ cup water. Stir and bring to boil covered for 5 minutes to thicken the sauce. Adjust the taste with salt and black pepper. Spoon the beef mixture into the baking dish and spread evenly. Sprinkle with mozzarella cheese. Bake in the oven for 15 minutes at 380 F until the cheese has melted and it's golden brown. Remove and cool for 4 minutes. Serve sprinkled with parsley.

Per serving: Cal 391; Fat 233g; Net Carbs 7.3g; Protein 20g

37. Spiralized Zucchini in Bolognese Sauce

Ingredients **for 4 servings**

4 zucchinis, spiralized

1 lb ground beef

2 bacon slices, chopped

2 garlic cloves

1 onion, chopped

1 tsp dried oregano

1 tsp sage

1 tsp rosemary

7 oz canned diced tomatoes

2 tbsp olive oil

Directions **and Total Time: approx. 35 minutes**

Cook the zoodles in warm olive oil over medium heat for 3-4 minutes and remove to a serving plate. To the same pan, add bacon, onion, and garlic and cook for 3 minutes. Add beef and cook until browned, about 4-5 minutes. Stir in the herbs and tomatoes. Cook for 15 minutes and serve over the zoodles.

Per serving: Cal 378; Fat 19g; Net Carbs 5.9g; Protein 41g

38.Juicy Beef with Rosemary & Thyme

Ingredients **for 4 servings**

2 garlic cloves, minced

2 tbsp butter

2 tbsp olive oil

1 tbsp rosemary, chopped

1 lb beef rump steak, sliced

Salt and black pepper to taste

1 shallot, chopped

½ cup heavy cream

½ cup beef stock

1 tbsp mustard

2 tsp soy sauce, sugar-free

2 tsp lemon juice

1 tsp xylitol

A sprig of rosemary

A sprig of thyme

Directions and Total Time: approx. 30 minutes

Set a pan to medium heat, warm in a tbsp of olive oil and stir in the shallot; cook for 3 minutes. Stir in the stock, soy sauce, xylitol, thyme sprig, cream, mustard and rosemary sprig, and cook for 8 minutes. Stir in butter, lemon juice, pepper and salt. Get rid of the rosemary and thyme. Set aside. In a bowl, combine the remaining oil with black pepper, garlic, rosemary, and salt. Toss in the beef to coat, and set aside for some minutes.

Heat a pan over medium-high heat, place in the beef steak, cook for 6 minutes, flipping halfway through; set aside and keep warm. Plate the beef slices, sprinkle over the sauce, and enjoy.

Per serving: Cal 411; Fat 31g; Net Carbs 4.6g; Protein 28g

39. Red Wine Beef Roast with Vegetable s

Ingredients **for 2 servings**

1 tbsp olive oil

1 lb brisket

½ cup carrots, peeled

1 red onion, quartered

2 stalks celery, cut into chunks

1 garlic clove, minced

Salt and black pepper to taste

1 bay leaf

1 tbsp fresh thyme, chopped

1 cup red wine

Directions **and Total Time: approx. 2 hours 20 minutes**

Season the brisket with salt and pepper. Brown the meat on both sides in warm olive oil over medium heat for 6-8 minutes.

Transfer to a deep casserole dish. Arrange the carrots, onion, garlic, thyme, celery, and bay leaf around the brisket and pour in the red wine and ½ cup of water. Cover the pot and place in the preheated to 370 F oven.

Cook for 2 hours. When ready, remove the casserole. Transfer the beef to a chopping board and cut it into thick slices. Top the beef with vegetables to serve.

Per serving: Cal 446; Fat 22g; Net Carbs 5.6g; Protein 52g

40. Grilled Steak with Green Bean s

Ingredients for 2 servings

2 rib-eye steaks

2 tbsp unsalted butter

1 tsp olive oil

½ cup green beans, sliced

Salt and black pepper to taste

1 tbsp fresh thyme, chopped

1 tbsp rosemary, chopped

1 tbsp fresh parsley, chopped

Directions and Total Time: approx. 20 minutes

Preheat a grill pan over high heat. Brush the steaks with olive oil and season with salt and black pepper. Cook the steaks for about 4 minutes per side; reserve. Steam the green beans for 3-4 minutes until tender.

Season with salt. Melt the butter in the pan and stir-fry the herbs for 1 minute; then mix in the green beans. Place over the steaks and serve. Enjoy!

Per serving: Cal 576; Fat 39g; Net Carbs 4.3g; Protein 51g

Seafood Recipes

41. Coconut Crab Patties

Preparation Time: **10 minutes**

Cooking time : 50 minutes

Servings **: 6**

Ingredients

- 2 tbsp coconut oil
- 1 tbsp lemon juice
- 1 cup lump crab meat
- 2 tsp Dijon mustard
- 1 egg, beaten
- 1 ½ tbsp coconut flour

Directions

1. In a bowl to the crabmeat, add all the ingredients, except for the oil; mix well to combine.

2. Make patties out of the mixture. Melt the coconut oil in a skillet over medium heat. Add the crab patties and cook for about 2-3 minutes per side.

Nutrition : Calories 277 - Fat 26.2g - Carbs 9g - Sugar 4g - Protein 7.5g – Cholesterol 31mg

42. Shrimp in Curry Sauce

Preparation Time **: 10 minutes**

Cooking time : 20 minutes

Servings **: 6**

Ingredients

- ½ ounce grated Parmesan cheese
- 1 egg, beaten
- ¼ tsp curry powder
- 2 tsp almond flour
- 12 shrimp, shelled
- 3 tbsp coconut oil
- Sauce
- 2 tbsp curry leaves
- 2 tbsp butter
- ½ onion, diced
- ½ cup heavy cream

- **½ ounce cheddar cheese, shredded**

Directions

1. Combine all dry ingredients for the batter.
2. Melt the coconut oil in a skillet over medium heat. Dip the shrimp in the egg first, and then coat with the dry mixture. Fry until golden and crispy.
3. In another skillet, melt butter.
4. Add onion and cook for 3 minutes.
5. Add curry leaves and cook for 30 seconds. Stir in heavy cream and cheddar and cook until thickened.
6. Add shrimp and coat well.
7. **Serve.**

Nutrition:

- Calories 190 at 16.3 g Carbohydrates 2.3 g
- Sugar 0.2 g Protein 8.7 g
- Cholesterol 52 mg

Smoothies

43. Berry Banana with Quinoa Smoothie

Preparation time: **10 minutes** Servings : **3**

Ingredients :

- ½ cup cooked quinoa, chilled 1 frozen banana
- 1 cup frozen raspberries or strawberries
- 1½ cups green tea, brewed and cooled ice cubes

Directions :

1. Place the quinoa, frozen banana sections, berries, and tea in the blender. Process until smooth. Serve.

Nutrition:

- Calories 146 Total Fat: 4.5 g Carbs: 23.5 g
- Sugars: 16.4 g
- Protein: 5.4 g

44. Vegan Sandwich with Tofu & Lettuce Slaw

- <u>Ingredients</u> **for 2 servings**

- ¼ lb firm tofu, sliced
- 2 low carb buns
- 1 tbsp olive oil

- Marinade
- 2 tbsp olive oil
- Salt and black pepper to taste
- 1 tsp allspice
- ½ tbsp xylitol
- 1 tsp thyme, chopped
- 1 habanero pepper, seeded and minced
- 2 green onions, thinly sliced
- 1 garlic clove

- Lettuce slaw
- ½ small iceberg lettuce, shredded
- ½ carrot, grated

- ½ red onion, grated
- 2 tsp liquid stevia
- 1 tbsp lemon juice
- 2 tbsp olive oil
- ½ tsp Dijon mustard
- Salt and black pepper to taste

- <u>Directions</u> **and Total Time: approx. 20 min + chilling time**
- In a food processor, blend the marinade ingredients for a minute. Pour the mixture over the tofu slices in a bowl. Place in the fridge to marinate for 1 hour. In a large bowl, whisk the lemon juice, stevia, olive oil, mustard, salt, and pepper. Stir in the lettuce, carrot, and onion; set aside.
- Heat 1 teaspoon of oil in a skillet over medium heat. Remove the tofu from the fridge and cook it for 6

minutes on all sides. Remove to a plate. Add the tofu to the buns and top with the slaw. Serve.

- **Per serving:** Cal 687; Fat 58g; Net Carbs 10.5g; Protein 23g

45. Grilled Cauliflower Steaks with Haricots Ver t

- <u>Ingredients</u> **for 2 servings**

- 1 head cauliflower, sliced lengthwise into 'steaks'

- 2 tbsp olive oil

- 2 tbsp chili sauce

- 1 tsp hot paprika

- 1 tsp oregano

- Salt and black pepper to taste

- 1 shallot, chopped

- 1 bunch haricots vert, trimmed

- 1 tbsp fresh lemon juice

- 1 tbsp cilantro, chopped

- <u>Directions</u> **and Total Time: approx. 30 minutes**

- Preheat grill to medium heat. Steam the haricots vert in salted water over medium heat for 6 minutes. Drain, remove to a bowl, and toss with lemon juice.

- In a bowl, mix the olive oil, chili sauce, hot paprika, and oregano. Brush the cauliflower steaks with the mixture. Place them on the grill, close the lid, and grill for 6 minutes. Flip the cauliflower and cook further for 6 minutes. Remove the grilled caulis to a plate; sprinkle with salt, black pepper, shallots, and cilantro. Serve with the steamed haricots vert.

- **Per serving:** Cal 234; Fat 16g; Net Carbs 8.4g; Protein 5.2g

46. Tofu & Vegetable Stir-Fry

- <u>Ingredients</u> **for 2 servings**

- 2 tbsp olive oil

- 1 ½ cups tofu, cubed

- 1 ½ tbsp flaxseed meal

- Salt and black pepper to taste

- 1 garlic clove, minced

- 1 tbsp soy sauce, sugar-free

- ½ head broccoli, cut into florets

- 1 tsp onion powder

- 1 cup mushrooms, sliced

- 1 tbsp sesame seeds

- <u>Directions</u> **and Total Time: approx. 15 min + chilling time**

- In a bowl, add onion powder, tofu, salt, soy sauce, black pepper, flaxseed, and garlic. Toss the mixture to coat and allow to marinate in the fridge for 20-30 minutes.

In a pan, warm the olive oil over medium heat. Add the broccoli, mushrooms, and tofu mixture and stir-fry for 6-8 minutes. Serve sprinkled with sesame seeds.

- **Per serving:** Cal 423; Fat 31g; Net Carbs 7.3g; Protein 25g

Sweets & Desserts Recipes

47. Chocolate Candies with Blueberries

Ingredients for 4 servings

2 cups raw cashew nuts

2 tbsp flax seed

1 ½ cups blueberry preserves, sugar-free

3 tbsp xylitol

10 oz unsweetened chocolate chips

3 tbsp olive oil

- **Instructions - Total Time**: around 6 minutes + cooling time
- Grind the cashew nuts and flax seeds in a blender for 50 seconds until smoothly crushed; add the blueberries and 2 tbsp of xylitol. Process further for 1 minute until well combined. Form 1-inch balls of the mixture. Line a baking sheet with parchment paper and place the balls on the baking sheet. Freeze for 1 hour or until firmed

up. In a microwave, melt the chocolate chips, oil and the remaining xylitol, for 95 seconds. Toss the truffles to coat in the chocolate mixture, put on the baking sheet, and freeze up for at least 3 hours.

- **Per serving**: Cal 253; Fat 18g; Net Carbs 4.1g; Protein 10g

48. Matcha Brownies with Macadamia Nuts

Ingredients for 4 servings

A pinch of salt

1 tbsp tea matcha powder

¼ cup coconut flour

¼ cup unsalted butter, melted

½ tsp baking powder

4 tbsp swerve confectioner's sugar

1 egg

½ cup chopped pistachios

- **Instructions - Total Time**: around 28 minutes
- Line a square baking dish with parchment paper and preheat the oven to 350 F. In a bowl, pour the melted butter, add swerve sugar and salt, and whisk to combine. Crack the egg into the bowl. Beat the mixture until the egg is incorporated. Pour the coconut flour, matcha and baking powder into a fine-mesh sieve and sift them into the egg bowl; stir. Stir in the pistachios

and pour the mixture into the baking dish to cook for 18 minutes. Remove and slice into brownie cubes.

- **Per serving**: Cal 243; Fat 22g; Net Carbs 4.3g; Protein 7.2g

49. Mascarpone & Strawberry Pudding

Ingredients for 6 servings

1 cup mascarpone, softened

2 oz fresh strawberries

1 ¼ cups coconut cream

1 tsp cinnamon powder

1 tsp vanilla extract

- **Instructions - Total Time**: around 25 minutes
- Put coconut cream into a bowl and whisk until a soft peak forms. Mix in vanilla and cinnamon. Lightly fold in mascarpone and refrigerate for 10 minutes to set. Spoon into serving glasses, top with the strawberries, and serve.
- **Per serving**: Cal 231; Fat 20g; Net Carbs 3g; Protein 6g

50. Dark Chocolate Brownies

Ingredients for 4 servings

10 tbsp butter

2 oz sugar-free dark chocolate

2 eggs, beaten

¼ cup cocoa powder

½ cup almond flour

½ tsp baking powder

½ cup erythritol

½ tsp vanilla extract

- **Instructions - Total Time**: around 30 min+ chilling time
- Preheat oven to 380 F. Line a baking sheet with parchment paper. In a bowl, mix cocoa powder, almond flour, baking powder, and erythritol until no lumps from the erythritol remain. In another bowl, add butter and dark chocolate and microwave both for 30 seconds. Mix the eggs and vanilla into the chocolate

mixture, then pour the mixture into the dry ingredients; mix well. Pour the batter onto the paper-lined sheet and bake for 20 minutes. Let cool completely and refrigerate for 2 hours. Slice into squares.

- **Per serving**: Cal 231; Net Carbs 3g; Fat 20g; Protein 4g

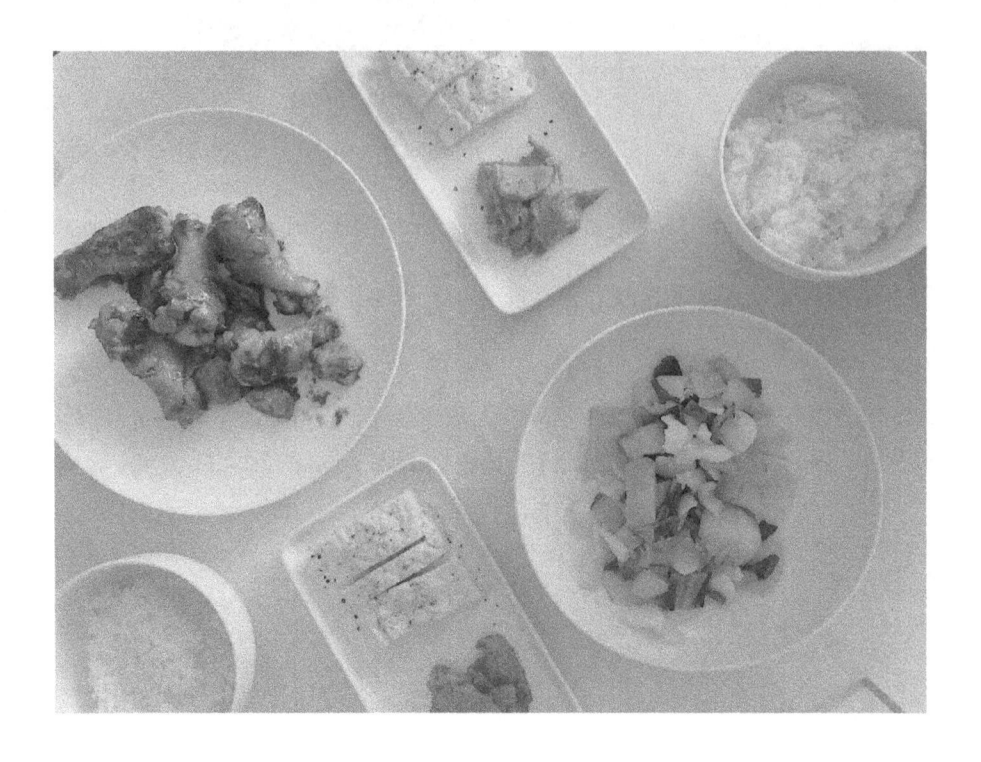

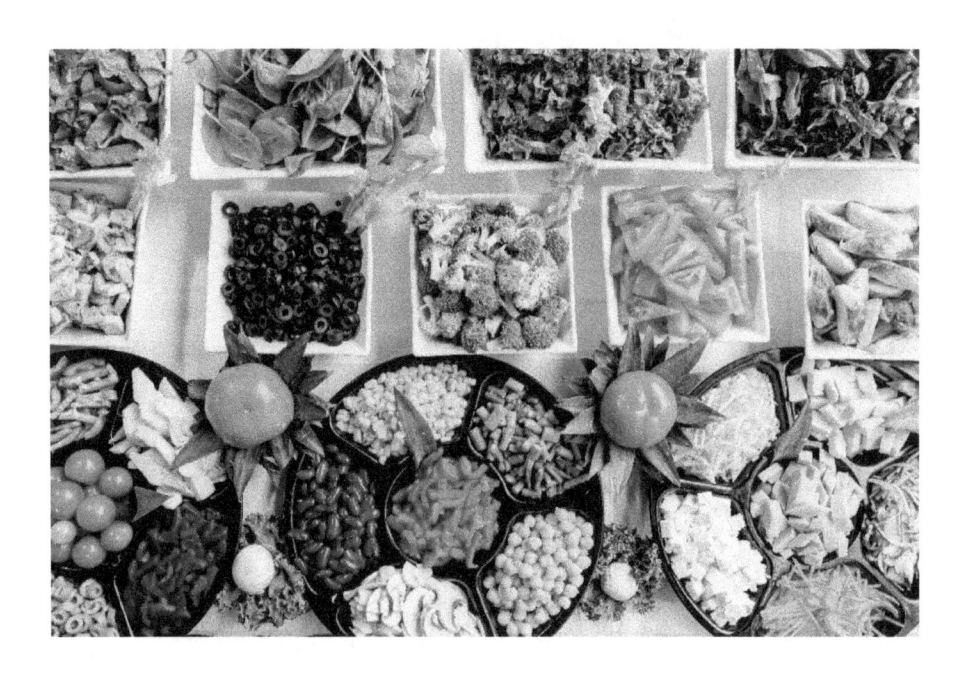

CONCLUSION

- ongratulations for making it this far! By now, I trust you already have a good understanding of the Ketogenic Diet and how it applies to you as you enjoy your 50s. Obviously, our goal here is to provide a Keto Diet guideline that works for you, taking into account your unique situation so that the best and most effective results can be achieved.
- The ketogenic diet is one that has many important aspects and information that you need to know as someone who wants to try this diet. It is important to remember the warning that we have given you at the beginning of the book that this is not a diet that is safe and that doctors don't recommend to try it, and if you are going to attempt it remember that you shouldn't do so for longer than six months and even then never without the constant supervision of a doctor or at the very least a doctor knowing that you're doing this and that you're following their guidelines and words to the letter so they can make sure you are safe.
- The ketogenic diet is a diet that believes that by minimizing your carbs while maximizing the good fat in your system while making sure that you're getting the protein you need; you will be happier and healthier. In this guidebook, we give you the information to know what this diet is all about, as well as describing the different types and areas that this diet will offer. Most people assume that there is only one way to do this and while there is one thing that the additional options share, there are four different options you can choose from. Each one has its unique benefits, and you should know about each type to learn what would be best for your body, which is why we have described them in the

- book for you to have the best information possible when you begin this diet for yourself.
- Another important thing about this diet is that many people don't understand the importance of exercise with this diet. The best way to become healthier is to do three things for yourself. Get the right amount of sleep, eat healthily, and make sure that you get the proper amount of exercise as well for your body to work at an optimum level. The exercises, such as the ones that we explained, are the best to go with your diet to make sure that you are getting the most out of it.
- For women who are on the go and have a busy lifestyle, we have provided recipes for a thirty-day meal plan so that you can make food quickly and have a great meal for their lifestyles. They also have enough servings for you to have leftovers so that you don't have to worry about preparing more food in the morning. Instead, you can simply pack it up and take it with you wherever you go. This works out so much easier for so many people because they don't have to cook in the morning, and it saves a busy person a lot of time.
- With all this information at your fingertips, you will be able to enjoy this diet and use it to your advantage. Another benefit that we offer is that we explain routines that you can do for yourself to make this diet last longer for you and to benefit your body better as a result. Routines are very important and can be a big help to your body but also your spirit and your mind. Good luck with your keto journey!
- One of the easiest ways to stay on your plan is to minimize the temptations. Remove the chocolate, candy, bread, pasta, rice, and sugary sodas you have supplied in your kitchen. If you live alone, this is an easy task. It is a bit more challenging if you have a family. The diet will also be useful for them if you plan your meals using the recipes included in this book.
- If you cheat, that must count also. It will be a reminder of your indulgence, but it will help keep you in line. Others may

believe you are obsessed with the plan, but it is your health and wellbeing that you are improving.

- When you go shopping for your ketogenic essentials be sure you take your new skills, a grocery list, and search the labels. Almost every food item in today's grocery store has a nutrition label. Be sure you read each of the ingredients to discover any hiding carbs to keep your ketosis in line. You will be glad you took the extra time.

- One significant motivation behind why we get so disappointed with standard weight control plans is that they regularly become misjudged and accomplish more damage than anything else.

- So, in case you're needing a little motivation to read the book again, simply don't be excessively hard on yourself on the off chance that you miss a class or enjoy somewhat more than you needed. With these statements, you will realize that disappointment is part to remember the procedure.

- But I think the most important thing I want you to learn from this book is this: it's never too late to make that change! It's never too late to try something new for self-improvement!